D1297569

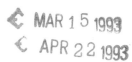

CHILDHOOD SCHIZOPHRENIA

CHILDHOOD SCHIZOPHRENIA

SHEILA CANTOR, M.D.
Medical Director
Schizophrenia Treatment and Research Foundation
of Manitoba

THE GUILFORD PRESS
New York   London

© 1988 The Guilford Press
A Division of Guilford Publications, Inc.
72 Spring Street, New York, NY   10012

Printed in the United States of America

Last digit is print number: 9 8 7 6 5 4 3 2 1

LIBRARY OF CONGRESS CATALOGING-IN-PUBLICATION DATA

Cantor, Sheila.
    Childhood schizophrenia / Sheila Cantor.
        p.   cm.
    Bibliography: p.
    Includes index.
    ISBN 0-89862-713-3
    1. Schizophrenia in children.   I. Title.
    [DNLM: 1. Schizophrenia, Childhood. WM 203 C232c]
RJ506.S3C36   1988
618.92′8982—dc19
DNLM/DLC
for Library of Congress   88-5180
                                   CIP

To Dr. Lauretta Bender and Dr. Barbara Fish
—the true pioneers in this most difficult field

Every generation has the privilege of standing on the shoulders of the generation that went before; but it has no right to pick the pockets of the first comer.
—Brander Matthews (1904), *Recreations of an Anthologist*

CONTENTS

CHILDHOOD
SCHIZOPHRENIA

INTRODUCTION

In July 1973, on the first day of my psychiatric residency, I met my first childhood schizophrenic, a 16-year-old girl whom I shall call "Megan." The chief resident introduced her to me as an "immature personality disorder," explaining to me that she had been admitted in an amnestic state, perplexed, and unable to recall the events of the 6 hours immediately prior to admission. The police had picked her up wandering on the streets uncertain of who she was or where she was going. The resident assured me that she was not psychotic and that the entire episode was, no doubt, a variant on an adolescent adjustment reaction.

Megan became my first psychotherapeutic case. In our sessions I experienced myself as being only slightly less perplexed than she was. I tried to explain my concern to my supervisor: I believed that if I pushed her at all she would decompensate into psychosis; he challenged me to do just that, assuring me that it was my own naiveté and inexperience that made me so fearful. I pushed her; she dropped out of therapy and returned to the hospital 8 months later floridly psychotic. In the next 15 months she began the arduous task of teaching me how to work with schizophrenic adolescents.

In January 1975 I found myself describing psychotherapy with Megan to Dr. Kalogerakis, a staff psychiatrist at Bellevue–NYU Medical Center. Dr. Kalogerakis responded with enthusiasm to my case description and apparently documented what he heard because when I arrived in July 1975 to do my Child and Adolescent Psychiatry Fellowship at Bellevue, "Marni" was assigned to me with these words: "Since you already have a working knowledge of how to treat adolescent schizophrenics, we will give you Marni, who is a severe borderline personality, and she will teach you how to work with borderlines."

Marni was also 16 years old when I met her. I accepted uncritically the idea that she was a severe borderline (she certainly was not displaying any symptoms I then recognized as arising from schizophrenic disease) and in desperation read and reread Otto Kernberg (1975) as I struggled to maintain a therapeutic alliance with this most disturbed young woman. Even when Marni described visual hallucinations and perceptual distortions, I interpreted these as hysterical phenomena, the result of her extreme suggestibility and the years of exposure to schizophrenic symptomatology during periods of hospitalization in Bellevue.

"Maria," the third childhood schizophrenic whom I encountered during my training years, was a 14-year-old girl from a family of schizophrenic individuals. She arrived at Bellevue mute and severely delusional (we learned when she finally talked). She introduced me to the school history of unidentified childhood schizophrenics, as her school records revealed a constant back-and-forth movement between special education and the regular classroom, beginning at age 6. Both the teachers at Bellevue and the psychologist found her fluctuating attention and capacity for learning quite remarkable.

"Mel" was a 6-year-old boy at whose case conference I received a formal introduction to the concept of childhood schizophrenia. Mel had been admitted to Bellevue Psychiatric Hospital for a diagnostic evaluation because he was already stressing existing treatment services. The formal thought disorder he demonstrated was very striking in one so young, but when I introduced him to my immediate supervisor I was told to diagnose him as an "overanxious reaction of childhood." Puzzled, I consulted with Dr. Campbell, another staff member on the children's unit. Dr. Campbell believed that the child was suffering from schizophrenia. This child was thus the subject of a diagnostic disagreement, and I therefore elected to present the boy to Dr. Theodore Shapiro at the Child Psychiatry Fellowship Seminar. At the end of the seminar Dr. Shapiro draped the child over his arm. The boy hung like a "floppy infant" while Dr. Shapiro remarked, "This is a Bender schizophrenic." I would never again fail to assess the motor tone of schizophrenic individuals.

BEAUTIFUL HANDICAPPED CHILDREN

> How unnatural! is an exclamation of pained surprise which some of the more striking instances of insanity in young children are apt to provoke. (Maudsley, 1880, p. 256)

The cases that I have described have a number of characteristics in common:

- All of these youngsters were attractive and appealing.
- On occasion all of these youngsters demonstrated normal functioning.
- All of these youngsters were hypotonic and had major deficits in motor, sensory, and cognitive functioning that intermittently severely compromised their ability to function.
- All of these youngsters perplexed mental health and education professionals, resulting in multiple evaluations and diagnoses, and failed interventions.
- All of these youngsters ultimately received a diagnosis of schizophrenia.

It is difficult for parents, teachers, and even mental health professionals to accept that a normal-appearing youngster, who after all still has years of development ahead, has a chronic and handicapping mental disorder. The prevailing difficulty with conceptualizing the brain as a biochemical and physiological organ encourages the persistence of magical hopes. "You really don't know, do you?" is a favorite invitation to practice denial and "hope for the best."

CHILDHOOD SCHIZOPHRENIA AS A DISTINCT SYNDROME

This book attempts to offer detailed descriptions of the manifestations of classical childhood schizophrenia, that is, schizophreniform disease from which those with a history of significant organic insult have been excluded. Detailed diagnostic scales are provided in the appendices, and information on the percentage of affected children who demonstrate a particular sign or symptom, as well as the stability of that particular symptom across age groups, is included in the text (Chapter 5).

This book reflects my own clinical bias: I believe that childhood schizophrenia deserves to be conceptualized as a distinct clinical syndrome, which is usually first manifest in prepubertal subjects but which can occur at any age (Cantor, Pearce, Pezzot-Pearce, & Evans, 1981). I believe this "syndrome" to be characterized by the primary symptoms of Bleuler (1911/1950) and to be complicated by moderate to severe sensory, motor, and cognitive deficits in functioning. I believe this syndrome to be the result of a dysfunctional cholinergic system (Cantor, 1980; Cantor, Trevenen, Postuma, Dueck, & Fjeldsted, 1980; Cantor et al., 1981). The hereditary component is prominent. The prognosis tends to be poor no matter what the age of onset, because the negative symptoms of schizophrenia predominate and because the disease process compromises normal development.

With few exceptions, those adults whom I have cared for who have demonstrated the signs of childhood schizophrenia have been extremely sensitive to phenothiazines; that is, if they respond at all, it is to low to moderate doses (a typical dose of fluphenazine in this type of patient would be an intramuscular injection of 6.25–12.5 mg every 2 weeks). I have encountered involuntary movements resembling tardive dyskinesia in a 20-year-old childhood schizophrenic who was medication-free (these movements were described in the literature of the 1920s, long before we had phenothiazines) and in several individuals who were on very low doses of medication or who had just begun pharmacotherapy. I have seen this often enough that I have grown wary of using phenothiazines in adult schizophrenics who demonstrate poor posture and poor muscle tone (although if the patient is floridly psychotic one has little choice).

FAMILY HISTORY

The stigma and denial that surround chronic mental illness are nowhere more evident than when one tries to obtain an accurate family history. Many families truly do not know of the existence of mentally ill relatives, since an aunt or an uncle who was institutionalized in childhood has often been forgotten by immediate relatives. Well-meaning grandparents frequently withhold information on mentally handicapped relatives in the hope that if this illness is never spoken of it can have no impact on future generations. Even when the parents of a schizophrenic child do know of the existence of a "funny" aunt or uncle, they are likely to withhold this information from the doctor in the hope that this will result in the doctor viewing their son or daughter more "objectively."

Table 1 gives detailed information on the families of 51 of the 54 subjects described in this book (no family history was available on 3 of the subjects). Denial is widespread, but many of the subjects have been known to me long enough so that "skeletons" have slowly emerged from family closets. Cases are listed only if they have been confirmed beyond a doubt. In some cases I have known a family for 2 or 3 years before an affected relative has been identified. (The derivation of "Group 1" and "Group 2" is explained in Chapter 5.) The coincidental prevalance of other neuropsychiatric disorders in these families (e.g., epilepsy, mental retardation, and speech delay) is noteworthy.

Some of the families are particularly hard hit. Although I have seen only 4 families in which more than one child is affected (and the 54 subjects described in this book are selected from 54 different families), in all 4 of these families one of the parents suffered from affective disease and the other parent manifested a schizophrenia-spectrum disorder. It is this combination that appears to be genetically the most malignant.

DEVELOPMENTAL DATA:
THE PARENT QUESTIONNAIRE

The developmental data in Chapters 2 to 4 have been derived from a detailed questionnaire (Appendix B); this was completed by 29 parents of schizophrenic children who were 10 years of age or younger when their parents completed the questionnaire, and by 64 parents of "normal" controls who were 6 years of age or younger when their parents completed the questionnaire. Most parents exercised great care in com-

Table 1
Family history

	Group 1		Group 2	
	N	%	N	%
Schizophrenia (chronic, hospitalized)	4/21	19	6/30	20
Schizophrenia spectrum disease (including schizotypal personality disorder)	7/21	33	12/30	40
Acute psychotic episode	4/21	19	6/30	20
Suicide	4/21	19	2/30	7
Epilepsy	2/21	10	2/30	7
Mental retardation	2/21	10	7/30	23
Speech delay	1/21	5	3/30	10
Alcoholism	3/21	14	10/30	33
No history of acute psychotic episode or schizophrenia	9/21	43	12/30	40
Total denial of any of the above	8/21	38	6/30	20
Member of social class IV or V[a]				
Mothers	10/17	59	19/23	83
Fathers	7/17	41	12/22	55
Member of social class I or II[a]				
Mothers	6/17	35	3/23	13
Fathers	8/17	47	7/22	32

Note. The derivation of Group 1 and Group 2 is explained in Chapter 5. No significant differences emerged between the two groups.

[a]Hollingshead and Redlich (1953).

pleting the questionnaires, frequently consulting with each other and checking diaries, which at least some of the families had maintained during the index child's infancy.

ACKNOWLEDGMENTS

I wish I had known, during the years when I was responsible for the treatment of Megan, Marni, Maria, and Mel, what I now know. Instead of psychodynamic interpretations, even those that were firmly reality based, I would have offered education designed to circumvent thought disorder, gross motor therapy designed to improve body concept, and an explanation of symptomatology designed to awaken and nurture a concept of self-regulation. Marni was truly harmed by my disbelief of her symptoms, and today she is a revolving-door patient at a state hospital facility (the same psychiatrist who once insisted that she was a "borderline personality disorder" now describes her as a "textbook paranoid schizophrenic"). In my heart, it is to her, and to all those who suffer from childhood schizophrenic disease, that this book is truly dedicated.

During the 9 years that schizophrenic children have been the subjects of intensive study at the University of Manitoba Medical Center, a number of investigators have made major contributions to this work: Dr. Jane Evans, a geneticist, collaborated in the development of the Physical Characteristic Scale; Drs. John Pearce and Terry Pezzot-Pearce are the clinical psychologists with whom the Symptom Scale was developed, and it was they who performed most of the WISC-R testing described in Chapter 6. Mr. Mohammed Inayatulla, a psychometrist, completed the WISC-R testing on our subjects after the Pearces left Winnipeg. Mr. Russell Dueck, an occupational therapist, assisted by Brenda Fjeldsted and Paula Villafana, performed all the motor assessments described in Chapter 6; and Drs. Dan Harper and Keith Wilson, both research psychologists, assisted by Mr. Kuldip Maini, performed all the statistical data analyses presented in this book. Maryanne Ashley, Bob Herzog, Wendy Walder, and Sharon Loggia are the treatment staff of the Schizophrenia Foundation who have played a major role in developing the treatment strategies and the strength/deficit assessment forms described in Chapter 7; and Ms. Constance Dureski is the graduate student who collected the data on the control children presented in Chapter 3.

The research described in this book was supported by a grant from the Manitoba Medical Services Foundation, Inc.

A Special Thank You

To those of my teachers whose dedication to teaching prodded (through opposition) and nurtured (with encouragement) my early attempts at conceptualization (in the order in which we met): Drs. Nahum Spinner, Nate Epstein, Wendell Watters, John Goodman, and Paul Grof at McMaster University; and Drs. Ted Shapiro, Natalie Yarrow, Stella Chess, Archie Silver, Peter Kim, and Mohine Hassibbi at Bellevue, I remain eternally grateful.

Thanks are also due to those of my colleagues who have provided the dialogue and encouragement needed to allow the ideas implanted during the student years to mature and develop (in the order in which we met): Drs. Clarice Kestenbaum, Richard Snyder, Cynthia Trevenen, Jane Evans, John Pearce, Terry Pezzot-Pearce, Nancy Roeske, Larry Silver, Joaquim Puig-Antich, Peter Tanguay, and Ludwik Szymanski.

Special thanks are due to the parents of schizophrenic children for the care that they have taken in documenting their child's behavior longitudinally and in providing detailed accounts to this investigator. Some families have been coming to my office for more than 9 years, despite the fact that I have "cured" none. Each developmental hurdle has been crossed by these families with a strength and a courage that are exemplary.

May this book help ensure that childhood schizophrenics will be identified, that the services they require will be developed, and that the future will bring rapid advances in our ability to understand and to treat this most disabling of disorders.

CHAPTER ONE

A HISTORICAL PERSPECTIVE

And surely our profession will in the future be able to apply its knowledge of brain function and development and the laws of heredity towards making the most of such lives, strengthening the weak points without forcing down the strong ones, saving from misery and ruin without depriving humanity of their originality and intenseness.—Clouston (1884, p. 258)

It is both humbling and exciting to discover these illuminating words written so long ago by the fathers of contemporary psychiatry. Humbling because our progress has been less dramatic than they expected, and exciting to encounter ourselves and our patients in accounts written more than 100 years ago.

Psychotic children are described in every major textbook on psychiatric disorders. They are neither the result of the stresses of contemporary living, nor have they been "cured" by the advances of medicine (although dementia should no longer complicate syphilis and phenylketonuria, nor should it be seen in association with Sydenham's chorea).

An excellent description of schizophrenia in children was published 55 years ago by Howard Potter (1933). Even though a diagnosis of schizophrenia was confirmed at the 30-year follow-up of Potter's subjects (Bennett & Klein, 1966), throughout the 1960s, '70s, and '80s controversy has raged over the validity of making a diagnosis of schizophrenia in childhood (Cantor, Evans, Pearce, & Pezzot-Pearce, 1982; Fish & Ritvo, 1979). In 1964 the British Working Group on Childhood Schizophrenia (Creak, 1964) proposed a definition of childhood schizophrenia that was both overinclusive (the traditional organic–functional dichotomy was abandoned) and far removed from Bleuler (1911/1950). This departure from classical psychiatry appears to have set the stage for the final denunciation of the concept of schizophrenia in children (Rutter, 1972). Childhood Schizophrenia was not recognized as a valid diagnosis by the *Diagnostic and Statistical Manual of Mental Disorders*, third edition (DSM-III; American Psychiatric Association, 1980), so that it became necessary to reaffirm its validity in the psychiatric literature (Cantor, 1982; Cantor *et al.*, 1982).

In an effort to better understand the apparent difficulties involved in conceptualizing schizophrenia in childhood, I have turned to the psychiatric literature. My training director had begun our course on childhood schizophrenia with Potter's 1933 paper. I wondered how physicians had described psychotic children before Potter.

THE 19TH CENTURY: "BADNESS" OR "MADNESS"?

Descriptions of "insanity in children" were scattered throughout the psychiatric literature of the 19th century, most authors carefully noting that such insanity was "rare" and placing emphasis instead on "vulnerability" and "diathesis." When all else failed and a child had to be declared depraved, morality was quickly invoked and parents were often apportioned the blame (Brierre de Boismont, 1857).

Thus, the reaction of Brierre de Boismont to two cases of "juvenile insanity" was abrupt and to the point: a 6-year-old child was described as "extremely difficult to manage," and a 10-year-old was described as becoming "more and more perverted" (A1).*

A thoughtful contemporary of Brierre de Boismont's, John Conolly (1861–1862), did recognize the importance of what would later be termed "functional psychosis":

> The occasional existence of a disordered state of the mental faculties in children, not depending on any temporary condition of an inflammatory kind, or on recognized chronic disease, and not on the result of accident, and more resembling mania than imbecility, does not seem to have been noticed even by Medical

---

*The actual quotations are provided in Appendix C. These are identified in the text by the letter "A" and the appropriate number.

Practitioners until somewhat recently, and certainly has not attracted particular attention. (p. 395)

Conolly expressed the hope that an enlightened society was ready to recognize that "the mind was an attribute of value in every human being" (A2). His clinical descriptions of disturbed children were remarkably detailed, including behavioral observations, descriptions of posture, descriptions of motility disorders, and observations on physiognomy (A3). Even children with lesser degrees of disturbance, who would now be regarded as personality disorders, were described in some detail by Conolly (A4). With the words "no juvenile peculiarity, or waywardness or violence, should induce despair," he pleaded for practical intervention and caring treatment (A5 and A6).

By the middle of the 19th century, J. Crichton Browne (1859–1860) had suggested that it was important to distinguish the various mental disorders of childhood from each other:

Dementia must be carefully distinguished from idiocy; in the latter case, mind is congenitally absent, and has never existed; whilst in the former, mind, having existed, is veiled and diseased. . . . Dementia may be recognised in its earlier stages by slight incoherence, and by a want of connexion of ideas. (p. 301)

Browne nevertheless shared the biases of the times; for example, he attributed disease to "moral insanity" and overvalued the importance of imaginary companions (which he regarded as hallucinations and the products of a "dangerously precocious" imagination).

Maudsley's (1890) *The Pathology of the Mind* included a full chapter devoted to the "Insanity of Early Life." Maudsley considered two broad categories of mental derangement in children: that characterized by mental excitement and attended by an incoherence of ideas, and that which he termed an "affective derangement." In the first category he included "choreic insanity, cataleptoid insanity, and epileptic insanity." The cases he described under cataleptoid insanity might well have been considered cases of childhood schizophrenia by Potter, Bradley, Kanner, Despert, Bender, or Creak:

Another form which insanity takes sometimes in childhood is that of a more or less complete ecstasy: . . . It generally occurs in young children. The little patient lies perhaps for hours or days seemingly in a kind of mystical abstraction, with limbs more or less rigid or fixed in strange postures; sometimes there is insensibility to impressions, while in other instances vague answers are given, or there is utterly incoherent raving with sudden outbursts of wild shrieks from time to time. (p. 272)

Case descriptions offered under the category "affective derangement" also sound familiar (A7). Maudsley divides "affective insanity" into "instinctive insanity" and "moral insanity," based upon his view that humanity is possessed of two inborn instincts: that of "self-conservation" and that of "propagation." Like his contemporaries, Maudsley regarded much of juvenile insanity as being due to a perversion of these instincts (A8 and A9).

The majority of the 19th-century journal articles on insanity in children consisted of isolated case reports. All of the authors seemed to agree (1) that insanity in children is rare, or at least that it seldom is brought to medical attention; (2) that "epilepsy is the most common nervous disease in children"; and (3) that insanity in children is more likely to "partake of the character of mental defect, and the majority of cases may be properly classed under the head of idiocy or imbecility."

A review article written by Harriet Alexander at the end of the 19th century suggested that physicians were beginning to think developmentally. The "weak inhibitions of the child" were appreciated and understood as the "foundation of terror and suspicion" (Alexander, 1893). The existence of vulnerable children, the "insane diathesis," had been well described and generally recognized by 1884 (Clouston). The concept was, however, being applied indiscriminately to both the gifted and the vulnerable.

According to Alexander, much "insanity" in children was regarded as "delirium rather than mania" (Alexander, 1893, quoting Maudsley and Clouston), and it was argued that delirium sets in at a lower temperature in the "sensitive" child:

Such children, independently of temperature, are subject to gusts of unreasonable elevation during which they are quite beside themselves, rushing about wildly, shouting, fighting, not really knowing what they are about; this coming on at intervals like the attacks of disease. (Clouston, as quoted by Alexander, 1893, p. 517)

On the subject of paranoia in children, Alexander's review article cited at least one author who insisted:

that the persecutional delusional paranoiac presents special characters in childhood. They are wild, unsociable, inclined to solitude and isolation, somber and taciturn, defiant and suspicious, living apart from their comrades, regarding these last as scoffers, and already interpreting to their disadvantage the most insignificant event. Such a delusional state may of course have the usual forensic results. (Pottier, as quoted by Alexander, 1893, p. 517)

1900–1920: SCHIZOPHRENIA IN ADULTS DEFINED

The early 20th-century literature gave the world Bleuler's and Kraepelin's detailed descriptions of dementia praecox. The "fathers" of the concept of dementia praecox and schizophrenia (Bleuler, 1911/1950; Kraepelin, 1919/1971) made only a few statements regarding insanity in the prepubertal child. Both agreed that the disease had certainly begun in childhood in a percentage of their patients (5% according to Bleuler and 3.5% according to Kraepelin). Both maintained that in a percentage of cases the disease could reduce the victim to feeblemindedness, idiocy, or imbecility, and that this was particularly likely to occur in early childhood. Those characteristics described by some authors as an "insane diathesis," "nervousness," "oversensitivity," "psychopathy" (discussed later), and so forth were regarded by Bleuler and Kraepelin as early signs that the schizophrenic process was already manifest.

Perhaps in response to Bleuler's and Kraepelin's descriptions of the gravity of mental disease, prevention began to be advocated in the psychiatric literature. Charles Holmes pleaded for psychiatrists to recognize that "it is equally important to know that premonitory symptoms of insidiously developing mental disease often occur during early childhood and go unrecognized," and he urged physicians to be on the alert

for "marked evidences of an abnormal degree of mental excita-
bility and suggestibility" (1912, p. 283).

The inability of the child to elaborate a delusional state
was described early in the 20th century:

> The insane child may suffer from maniacal outbursts, emotional
> or intellectual depression, hallucinations, transitory delusions,
> obsessions and imperative impulses, and he may, of course,
> from the violence of the disease, be left demented or imbecile,
> but he cannot present the rich growth of delusions shown by
> his elder brother. He who has never heard of kings can not have
> the delusions that he is a king, and only those who have had
> strongly impressed upon them the dogma of the unpardonable
> sin can believe they have committed it. He alone can think he is
> persecuted who has learned something of the real persecutions
> that exist in the world. The child cannot show the curious
> perversions of logic of the adult paranoiac because logic itself is
> only just beginning to appear in him. (Burr, 1905, p. 36)

Although several vivid clinical descriptions of psychotic
children were published between 1905 and 1910 (De Sanctis,
1906; Heller, 1905, 1908; Vogt, 1909; Weygandt, 1906 [see
Lay, 1938]), the majority of psychiatrists continued to "lump"
severely demented children with amented children, as no criteria were suggested for the diagnosis of psychosis in children.

Case studies of "atypical children" also continued to appear in the literature, and the tendency to be concerned about
both the gifted and the defective persisted (Goodhart, 1913).
Goodhart believed that gifted children could be allowed to
develop their special skills, provided that great care was taken
not to "allow their emotions to become unduly awakened." He
maintained that "the basic radical of the true juvenile psychosis is an internal strife—an inadequacy in the reasoning faculties and judgement."

The Youthful Psychopath:
The Vulnerable Child Defined

Detailed descriptions of children described as "youthful
psychopaths" were published by Courtney in 1911. These
descriptions included a distinctive "bodily habit" and "slender

musculature, a narrow chest, scaphoid scapulae, drooping shoulders" as well as descriptions of "a vascular hypotonicity, with the vasomotor ataxia which so commonly accompanies this last-mentioned condition."

Courtney further described such a child as:

[having] vivid dreams . . . it will toss and tumble about the bed all through the night, grind its teeth, cry out loud or from time to time mumble disjointed phrases. . . . the morbid emotionalism of this child overshadows its intellectuality, shapes its character and compels its thought and action. . . . in the youthful psychopath fear is the emotion that dominates all cerebral activity . . . [leading to] pallor, cries, palpitation of the heart, muscular trembling and relaxation of the sphincters . . . [as well as] tics. . . . (1911, p. 220)

The "psychopathic child" was described as being "shy and diffident" with strangers but "self-willed and domineering" in the home. Courtney anticipated the ego psychologists when he described this child's "great difficulty with inhibition" which manifested itself as a "serious lack of self-control."

Courtney advocated that the diet of psychopathic children be controlled, limiting intake to food that was nutritious and "easy of digestion and assimilation, and inconsiderable in waste." He also stressed the importance of correcting faulty postural habits, of "nipping in the bud of anti-social tendencies," and of providing good role models.

A contemporary paper by Farnell (1914) described the "psychopathic child" in somewhat more vague terms, although Farnell too argued for the importance of prevention. He too worried about:

poor sleep in the child, frightening dreams, nervous restlessness at night, variability in mood, headaches . . . and "bad habits," such as nail biting, bed-wetting, facial tics, fits of temper, oversensitiveness at the sight of suffering, and the seeing of evil in the innocent enjoyments of life. (1914, p. 685)

The children whom Farnell described were less homogeneous than those described by Courtney, although these children too were very disturbed and had first-degree relatives afflicted with alcoholism, epilepsy, and mental retardation.

Farnell's paper even included an excellent description of a child who was the victim of incest, and he described the severe distortion in the development of the child's personality which followed the incident.

Farnell left the description of the "psychopathic child" quite abruptly to describe the "model child":

> a child who lacks affection . . . [displays] uninterestedness in work at school, absence of desire to play, inattention, idleness, fearfulness, irritability . . . [is] dreamy . . . [and has] evident difficulty with sex problem. (1914, p. 687)

He described two children with this "shut-in" type of personality, documenting in each case the slow development of dementia praecox.

Farnell attempted to explain these two different types of pathological personality, the "psychopathic" and the "shut-in," as being related to a differential response to internal and external stimuli: Emotion in the psychopath bears a close relation to external stimuli; whereas in predementia praecox, emotion bears close relation to internal stimuli. He argued for the creation of a hospital school which would be capable of "directing and modifying" the development of disturbed children.

1920–1929: A TIME FOR FIRSTS

The decade from 1920 to 1929 included many "firsts" in the literature on childhood psychosis: the first report of standardized testing (Goddard, 1920), the first detailed description of treatment (Witmer, 1920), the first retrospective chart study (Strecker, 1921), the first "high-risk" study (Canavan & Clark, 1923a, 1923b), and the first attempt at a large-scale epidemiologic study (Hyde, 1922–1923).

In 1920 a population of insane children, at the Concord Asylum for the Insane, was examined by an assistant from the Vineland Laboratories (Goddard, 1920). The analysis of the results revealed peculiarities that have come to be regarded as typical of childhood schizophrenia (even though the tests were performed on children then regarded as "juvenile psychopaths"):

Whereas the normal child or the feeble-minded reaches his level by answering all the questions as they come, up to almost his final stopping point, the insane scatter, i.e., their failures are scattered through several years and are found side by side with their successes. (Goddard, 1920, p. 512)

The psychopath gives peculiar and individual reactions instead of those which one would expect. He is apt to fall in to the use of nonsense syllables when giving 60 words in three minutes. He interpolates peculiar things in reading. He uses many-syllabled words in the places where the ordinary child uses simple words. (pp. 513–514)

In describing the reaction of the children, Goddard reported a "number of indications of perseveration, automatism, sound associations, repetition of stimulus words, etc."

Further descriptions of these "psychopathic children" were provided by Goddard (A10), who concluded that "little is known as to the prognosis and treatment" (A11).

The first detailed case history of the treatment of a preschool psychotic child was published in 1920 by Lightner Witmer (A12). Witmer said of the child: "he has no desires except to be let alone." The boy's parents had brought him to be educated, and the details regarding the way in which this was accomplished are the real subject of this paper. The child's facility with form boards and with rote learning is documented, as are his passivity ("and even now he will never dress himself if he can get somebody else to do it for him"), his tendency to reproduce the exact intonation of those who were teaching him, his tendency to perseverate (which his teacher mistook for "persistent concentration"), and his extreme fearfulness.

In 1921 Edward Strecker published the first retrospective chart study on the subject of childhood psychosis. Strecker reviewed 5,000 consecutive hospital admissions to a state hospital, reporting that, in his view, there were only 18 undoubted psychoses in children under the age of 15 among these 5,000 admissions. He declared that he had "carefully searched for" cases of dementia praecox and found only four cases. He concluded that this rarity of cases of dementia praecox among the young was "more than accidental." He did, however, admit that he excluded from his statistics "psychotic manifestations or episodes in epileptics, constitutional psychopaths, psychoneurotics, or the mentally defective." In this paper we have the first documented insistence that children with schizophrenia must present exactly like adults with schizophrenia, and that the disease must arise *de novo* in a previously healthy individual and result in a deterioration from a previous level of functioning.

The first high-risk study (i.e., the first study of the children of diagnosed schizophrenics) was published by Myrtelle Canavan and Rosamond Clark in the early 1920s (Canavan & Clark, 1923a). The study had many limitations, freely acknowledged by the authors, the most serious of which was that at the time the study was published 52% of the offspring were less than 10 years of age (well below the teenage years when the majority of schizophrenics are identified). Perhaps the most interesting aspect of the study was that it found a significant number of the children of schizophrenics were manifesting conduct disorders (7.8% of the children of schizophrenics were judged to be conduct disorders compared with only 1.4% of the children in the control group). The authors suggested that this could be due to a lack of home control.

The first epidemiologic study, which attempted to determine the prevalence rate of major psychiatric disturbances in children, was performed at the instigation of Hyde, in the state of Utah. A massive testing program of schoolchildren attempted to identify "feeble-minded" and "prepsychotic" children (Hyde, 1922–1923). The study utilized 20 university students, who were majoring in psychology, to test over 15,000 children. The study found that although the number of retarded children decreased rapidly from the lower to the higher grades, the "nervous" and "excitable" children were equally distributed across grade levels. The study concluded that "1% of the children examined were nervous, restless and excitable and therefore unstable."

Hyde postulated that "as the instructions became longer and more complex they could not be held in the attention of the nervous child sufficiently long for the problem to be completed, therefore, the child became confused and failed in the test" (1922–1923, p. 45). He hoped that this study would result in psychiatric social workers being introduced into the school who would "follow the individual nervous children into their homes and all other environment, and their work can be of the greatest value in preventing the nervous and unstable child from becoming the psychotic adult" (p. 48). With this paper, Hyde thus anticipated the child guidance movement.

A number of papers appeared in the 1920s that claimed to be providing detailed clinical descriptions of psychosis in "children" (Burr, 1925, Kasanin & Kaufman, 1929). In all cases, the authors dated the onset of dementia praecox to the time of puberty and provided very little information on the child's infancy and early childhood. Two biases were becoming very evident in the literature: (1) schizophrenia was equated with dementia—if the patient recovered or did well the diagnosis was changed (Kasanin & Kaufman 1929); and (2) schizophrenia was not recognized in young children—as authors continued to say that "mania is the insanity of early childhood" (Burr, 1925). Lethargic and catatonic schizophrenic children continued to be lost to "feeblemindedness" (Witmer, 1920; see section "Childhood Schizophrenia or Mental Retardation," later in this chapter). The one exception to this was "original paranoia," which was again clearly described:

> The parents notice that, even as a child, their son is unlike the other children in the family. . . . he has already become asocial. He is friendless, or has one or two boy friends, with whom alone he plays. He is selfish and never really learns the boys' code of honor and behavior. Often he is precocious and reads books beyond his comprehension, while failing in his school lessons. Before puberty, he loses, he may never have shown it, affection for his parents . . . and the first signs of what will later develop into delusions of persecution appear. That is to say, he begins to have a feeling that he is not being treated justly, his little world is against him. (Burr, 1925, p. 160)

1930–1939: A BEGINNING IS MADE

During the decade from 1930 to 1939, the effort to conceptualize exactly what was meant by schizophrenia in childhood became intense and more focused. The development of "acute care" psychiatric facilities for children provided trained child psychiatrists with an opportunity to observe children who were psychotic but not yet demented (Lurie, Tietz, & Hertzman, 1936; Potter, 1933); an attempt was made to define the "schizoid" personality (Childers, 1931); the first retrospective, developmental studies of adult schizophrenics were published (Bowman & Kasanin, 1933; Kasanin & Veo, 1932); and a thoughtful effort was made to differentiate the psychoses of childhood (Heller, 1930; Lay, 1938).

The decade began with a paper by Theodor Heller (1930) in which he argued for the differentiation of the syndrome that bears his name from dementia praecox (for this historical review Wilfred C. Hulse's 1954 translation of Heller's paper was used). To illustrate his point, Heller provided a detailed case description of "the only case of schizophrenia" he had ever diagnosed in a child (A13), insisting that "this early form of schizophrenia is entirely different in its course from the cases of dementia infantilis [Heller's syndrome] which have been observed until now." Beyond making this statement, Heller seemed to believe that the case spoke for itself and offered no other convincing argument.

A detailed description of a group of children whom he termed "schizoid" was published by A. Childers in 1931. This appears to have been the first published study describing children thus identified:

> Attention is directed to a particular type of problem child which we have termed "schizoid," not only for lack of a better term, but because the symptoms resemble those usually regarded as characteristic of the early stages of schizophrenia. (1931, p. 106)

The case descriptions are indeed interesting. They include descriptions of behavioral disturbances ("wastes time of whole class"), teacher reaction ("'queer' conduct rather than 'wrong' conduct"), developmental history ("walking and talking were somewhat delayed"), sleep disturbance ("he talks a good deal in his sleep"), and psychotic manifestations (" in class he would suddenly laugh aloud for no apparent reason . . . he talks to himself and annoys others").

Childers described the efforts of both teachers and classmates to help (A14), and followed each detailed case description with a discussion (A15). He concluded:

We believe that in cases of this type we are dealing with serious mental illness in the making. Many such children as these here described, unless their lives are radically changed, will in due time become the psychotics of adulthood. The psychosis will very likely be a schizophrenia. (p. 133)

Howard Potter's classic paper "Schizophrenia in Children" appeared in 1933. Stressing the difference between children and adults (A16), Potter presented a set of criteria for making the diagnosis of schizophrenia in the prepubertal child:

For purposes of clarity, the term "schizophrenia" in this communication is limited to such reaction types as are characterized by:

1. A generalized retraction of interests from the environment.
2. Dereistic thinking, feeling and acting.
3. Disturbances of thought, manifest through blocking, symbolization, condensation, perseveration, incoherence and diminution sometimes to the extent of mutism.
4. Defect in emotional rapport.
5. Diminution, rigidity and distortion of affect.
6. Alterations of behavior with either an increase of motility leading to incessant activity, or a diminution of motility, leading to complete immobility or bizarre behavior with a tendency to perseveration or stereotypy. (1933, p. 1254)

Six detailed case histories were provided by Potter (A17). In all cases he was careful to search for "organicity" and to exclude questionable cases. He concluded his paper with the comment:

There is a superficial resemblance of schizophrenic children to certain so-called unstable mental defectives. The schizophrenic child often appears mentally deficient because the libido is invested with the patient himself, thus interfering with the objectification of the intellectual processes. It is the thought of the writer that a careful psychiatric study, from a psychodynamic approach, of the patients in institutions for mental defectives, might demonstrate that schizophrenia in children is not as rare as is now generally believed. (p. 1268)

The first retrospective developmental study of adult schizophrenics was a study that attempted to reconstruct the school histories of a group of inpatients who had been confined to the Boston Psychopathic Hospital (Kasanin & Veo, 1932). These investigators traced the school histories of 54 adult psychotics, being careful to exclude those in whom there was a question of mental deficiency.

Kasanin and Veo divided their patients into five groups, reporting that one half of the psychoses had developed in adults who were classified as either Group I ("odd" children) or Group V ("nobodies"). In the other half of their cases, "the psychoses could not have been foreseen or anticipated" (A18 and A19).

Kasanin (Bowman & Kasanin, 1933) followed this initial retrospective study with a multidimensional study of schizophrenic individuals that, in some aspects, anticipated the multiaxial approach to diagnosis adopted by the American Psychiatric Association's (1980) DSM-III. Ten etiological factors, which were regarded as significant, were "coded for" in 151 patients. The group of psychiatrists who did the coding attempted to "code cases on the basis of what was shown in the actual record of the case" (i.e., this study too was a retrospective chart study). The authors cautioned that "our figures are nothing more than individual opinion and we make no pretense of omniscience or infallibility."

In all, 126 cases were coded as having two or more causes:

> The most frequently coded item under causation was environmental stress (81.4%), heredity was second (64.3%). Constitutional anomalies—mental, was third with a figure of 40.4%. (Bowman & Kasanin, 1933, p. 647)

> . . .These twelve cases might be said to represent the pure cases of "constitutional schizophrenia." (p. 648)

> We would say a typical case of this type would be one in which there was a definite family history of mental disease, especially of schizophrenia. The individual from very early childhood would be regarded as different, queer, or odd by those with whom he associated. He would seldom mix well with others. This oddity in personality would increase with the age of the patient. . . . The psychosis itself would be to a large extent an exaggeration of the peculiar type of personality which the individual had shown since early childhood. (p. 649)

In 1933 the second high-risk study of children of schizophrenics was published by Lampron. This study improved upon the Canavan and Clark (1923a) study in that 78% of the offspring of schizophrenics were older than 15 years at the time of the study. This paper for the first time acknowledged the stigma that is attached to mental disease:

> Because of the popular stigma attached to mental disease, with its attendant suggestion of hereditary influence, it was considered unwise to attempt to get into touch with all employers, teachers, and friends, for fear of hurting the standing of the individual in the community. (Lampron, 1933, p. 83)

The data were therefore limited to the offspring of only 75 matings.

The most significant findings in this study were that "38 individuals (20%) [were] reported to be suffering major forms of maladjustment" (these included psychoses, mental deficiency, psychotic predisposition, marked emotional instability, recurring simple depression, sexual delinquency, suicides, and murder); and that "18 individuals (10%) [were] reported to be suffering from minor forms of maladjustment" (these included seclusiveness, fear of mental disease, and neurotic traits).

Lampron summarized:

> Of the 186 offspring, 56, or 30%, suffer from either major or minor maladjustments manifested by varying degrees of personality deviation or antisocial behavior. . . . Thirty-eight, or 50% of the families investigated had from one to four children either mentally or socially maladjusted. (1933, p. 89)

In 1936 trained workers in child psychiatry reported, for the first time, on the prevalence rate of "functional psychoses" in an acute-care child psychiatric inpatient facility (Lurie et al., 1936). Other studies had reported on state hospital populations (Strecker, 1921: 18 cases in a population of 5,000) or "habit clinics" (Kasanin & Kaufman, 1929: 10 cases in an outpatient setting).

Twenty of the first 1,000 admissions to the Child Guidance Home in Cincinnati could be classified as psychotic. Only two of these 20 children had been referred because of a suspicion of mental disease, and only two of these children had been referred for observation by the parents themselves, "despite the fact that the children's behavior must have been very unusual." Other reasons for referral included "peculiar conduct" (nine cases), "determination of mental status" (two cases), "delinquency" (six cases), and "inability to adjust" (two cases).

Following the classification system of the American Psychiatric Association that was current at the time, 13 of the psychotic children were diagnosed as schizophrenic, six as psychopathic personality with psychosis, and one as psychotic with probable organic disease (a history of a possible attack of encephalitis was obtained in this case).

Six of the 13 schizophrenics showed impairment in all three spheres: intellectual, emotional, and social. Fifteen non-psychotic children also showed such impairment. Of these 15, 11 were mentally retarded, two had suffered from acute epidemic encephalitis, one had syphilis, and one was a psychopathic personality. Lurie *et al.* warned:

> It would seem fair to say that any child who is not mentally retarded and who has no organic involvement of the nervous system, but who shows a simultaneous break in the normal progression of its intellectual, emotional, and social development, is likely to develop a psychosis later in life and hence should be carefully watched. (1936, p. 1174)

The psychiatric findings in this study included the following:

> All the children showed disturbances of behavior, mood, insight and judgement. Stream of thought was abnormal in 12 children, 10 of whom were schizophrenic. . . . Sixteen of the series had delusions and 10 had hallucinations. . . . none of these children were disoriented. (pp. 1175–1176)

In conclusion, the authors reported that the children in this series had been followed for periods ranging from 1 to 13 years: "Nine of these children are now in Longview State Hospital, 1 in the State Institution for the Feebleminded, 1 in a correctional institution, and 2 are unaccounted" (p. 1176).

Finally, the decade that began with Heller ended with the review of "Schizophrenia-like Psychoses in Young Children" by R. Lay (1938). Lay reviewed many of the papers that have already been discussed in this historical perspective, including those by Kraepelin, Strecker, Kasanin and Kaufman, and Lurie *et al.*; and he noted the controversy over whether schizophrenia-like psychoses were as rare as many authors claimed.

Lay speculated that many cases might "exist in institutions for the feeble-minded," citing Potter's paper for advocating this view. He wondered if there was a tendency on the part of physicians, "when a severely abnormal child is brought for examination, to disregard parental statements that early development was normal" (p. 106).

Lay's paper contains a lengthy discussion of the differences and similarities between the forms of psychosis occurring in infants and young children. The discussion is thoughtful and comprehensive (A20). It anticipated the claim made by Fish and Ritvo in their comprehensive literature review (1979) that a great deal of the confusion in childhood psychosis stems from the abandonment of the traditional dichotomy between the "organic" and the "functional." Lay (1938) stressed that:

> Diagnosis should thus in general depend on the total picture, the reaction of the personality as a whole. (p. 127)

> Differentiation of the infantile psychoses from each other is still very much a matter of dispute. Dementia infantilis differs from hebephrenia in its more acute onset, more rapid progress and earlier age-incidence. Speech disturbance occurs earlier and is much more striking. Grebelskaja-Albatz . . . found among 22 schizophrenics poor motor coordination, lack of mime, clumsiness of gait and lack of poise. These contrast with the findings in dementia infantilis, in which motor activity is remarkably well preserved. (p. 129)

Lay's conclusion anticipated DSM-III:

> Dementia praecocissima (de Sanctis) and prepubertal schizophrenia show similar features to the schizophrenia of adults, as regards symptomatology and outcome. Dementia infantilis, first described by Weygandt and Heller, runs a somewhat acute course, leading to permanent dementia and loss of speech in a

few months. It is probably a separate clinical entity of organic aetiology. (p. 130)

While these controversies raged in psychiatry, "child psychiatry" was coming of age. By the end of the 30s, four giant figures in the field of childhood insanity were already making their observations and—in at least two instances—had begun publishing their observations: Leo Kanner published a first textbook for child psychiatry in 1935, and J. Louise Despert described her first cases of childhood schizophrenia in 1938. Bender and Bradley were, by this time, documenting their observations of schizophrenic children. The stage was set for the 1940s.

1940-1955: THE "DECADE OF THE CHILDHOOD PSYCHOTIC"

The Signs and Symptoms of Childhood Schizophrenia

The "decade of the childhood psychotic" was begun by J. Louise Despert in 1940 with "A Comparative Study of Thinking in Schizophrenic Children and in Children of Preschool Age." Despert objected to the fact that many writers had stressed "analogies between the [normal] child and the adult schizophrenic in their attitudes toward the world of reality." In agreement with the observations of Cameron (1938), she believed that in schizophrenia there was "a specific disorganization of thinking." Thus, Despert expressed concern that:

> The concept that schizophrenia represents a regression, from the point of view of thinking, in this instance, is based on two assumptions: that the child's thinking is fundamentally different from that of the adult; and furthermore, that in this psychosis, through some pathological process, a reversal to the earlier level of functioning takes place. (1940, p. 190)

Recognizing the implications of this hypothesis, Despert asked:

> Does the child at an early age experience illusions, misinterpretations, hallucinations, ideas of reference and influence, and other characteristic defects of perception and thinking in any

way comparable to those observed in the schizophrenic? When he plays and indulges in phantasy, does he lose contact with reality, even temporarily, as the schizophrenic is known to do? (p. 190)

In an effort to answer some of these questions, Despert studied 19 normal preschoolers, aged 1 year, 11 months to 5 years, 3 months, and compared their play behavior to that of 3 psychotic girls, aged 8 years, 6 months; 13 years, 4 months; and 8 years, 4 months. She concluded: "It is not possible to demonstrate in normal children true delusions and hallucinations or disorders characteristic of schizophrenic thinking" (1940, p. 211).

The clinical descriptions in this paper are rich (A21). Despert offered one "surprising" observation, as she noted that the most imaginative child was also the child who most frequently asserted that her play was fantasy (A22).

Despert's view of childhood schizophrenia (1938, 1947) was quite different in emphasis from that of Potter. She divided her cases into "acute" and "insidious," believing the prognosis to be worse in the "acute" forms* while acknowledging that there was not always an easy demarcation between the two presentations. She anticipated Kanner in placing emphasis upon "the inability of the schizophrenic child to tie up emotionally with people in his environment." Considering this inability to be "pathognomonic," she believed that "schizophrenia, whether of adult or child, is fundamentally a disturbance of affective contact."

Despert described the shizophrenic child's "excessive dependence on the mother or mother substitute." With no concern for any apparent contradiction,† she declared this to be of a "different nature than the dependence observed in neurotic or immature children."

Despert also described the "bizarre behavior" that she regarded as characteristic of the schizophrenic child, referring

*Author's note: Could the "acute" form be dementia infantilis?

†Many a pediatrician has insisted that this dependence of the child upon his or her mother signifies affective contact and that schizophrenia therefore does not occur in children.

to a lack of what she called "facetiousness" (A23) and a lack of "conformism" (A24), two characteristics of schizophrenic children that would now be referred to as "concrete thinking" and "oppositional behavior."

Despert's descriptions of the language of schizophrenic children have been considered by some as her most significant contribution to an understanding of childhood schizophrenia (this aspect is certainly the most frequently quoted). In addition to the tendency to formulate neologisms and a "peculiarity of speech" (A25), Despert described "a tendency to dissociate sign from function in their use of language. They have an exaggerated, often obsessive interest in word forms—detached from the emotional and intellectual content which these forms normally carry" (1947, p. 685).

Charles Bradley's monograph *Schizophrenia in Childhood* was published in 1941. In a later paper that summarized his views, Bradley (1947) stated:

> The reactions of mentally ill children can be properly evaluated only in terms of what is anticipated for most children of similar age and maturity, and no single standard scale of normality covers the entire childhood period. (p. 529)

Bradley carried out his studies of schizophrenic children at the Emma Pendleton Bradley Home, a children's psychiatric hospital. Fourteen of the 138 "maladjusted" boys and girls, who had been admitted "over a period of years," were judged to be schizophrenic (A26). Eight major behavioral characteristics were found to be especially prominent in these 14 children (Bradley's [1947, pp. 531–532] definitions of these characteristics are provided in parentheses):

1. Seclusiveness ("is considered as a strong tendency to consistently remain aloof from the society of other children").
2. Irritability when seclusiveness was disturbed ("is considered to be a reaction of anger when the seclusive activities are interrupted").
3. Daydreaming ("may be termed preoccupation with thoughts and fantasies definitely beyond what is usually noted in children of similar age and development").

4. Bizarre behavior ("is made up of actions and activities decidedly incongruous to the surroundings in which they occur. It includes such phenomena as posturizing, repetitive purposeless motions, unintelligible language, and irrelevant expression of emotion.").

5. Diminution of personal interests ("there are conspicuously fewer objects and activities toward which the child is attracted than one usually anticipates for most children of similar age and intelligence").

6. Regressive nature of personal interests.

7. Sensitivity to comment and criticism ("this includes both praise and blame").

8. Physical inactivity.

Bradley searched through 15 years of records at the Bradley Home to obtain data on the "age of earliest noted maladjustment." He found that in 29 out of the 32 children whose case records contained pertinent information there was evidence of maladjustment prior to 2 years of age. Twelve children were reported to show a lack of interest in their surroundings, particularly in other persons. Fourteen children gave some evidence of disturbed speech development. Nine children had presented feeding problems of various sorts, and motility disorders were distinctly recalled by the parents of 6 children. Bradley concludes:

> If both the history and symptoms suggest extreme seclusive tendencies in combination with several of the other eight traits that have been described, and are supported by a story of maladjustment going back into earliest childhood years, the possibility of schizophrenia must be considered and more complete psychiatric study is advised. (1947, p. 538)

In the tradition of Adolf Meyer (1908), Bradley believed that schizophrenia in childhood implied that there was an "inability to meet the demands of life even in infancy [which] suggests that a constitutional predisposition is the basic handicap." Bradley may well have helped to prepare the way for abandoning the traditional organic/functional dichotomy (Creak, 1964; Wing, 1985) by maintaining that:

schizophrenia in children appears to be a way of life rather than a disease, its existence is not incompatible with that of other handicaps such as mental deficiency, epilepsy, or cerebral palsy, to mention only a few coexisting conditions. (1947, p. 539)

Leo Kanner's historic paper was published in 1943. For this historical perspective I shall rely on Kanner's own assessment of his work (Kanner, 1949).

By 1949 Kanner had seen 50 children whom he referred to as "early infantile autism." In his view, the "characteristic features" of this diagnostic entity consisted of:

a profound withdrawal from contact with people, an obsessive desire for the preservation of sameness, a skillful and even affectionate relation to objects, the retention of an intelligent and pensive physiognomy, and either mutism or the kind of language which does not seem intended to serve the purpose of interpersonal communication. (1949, p. 416)

Kanner had been careful to exclude organicity (A27). His belief that functional psychosis should be separated from organic psychosis is made explicit by his discussion of the difference between infantile autism and Heller's disease (A28). He also insisted that autistics could be differentiated from congenital word deafness without too much difficulty (A29), and, in agreement with Despert (A30), he argued that:

The extreme emotional isolation from other people, which is the foremost characteristic of early infantile autism, bears so close a resemblance to schizophrenic withdrawal that the relationship between the two conditions deserves serious consideration. (p. 418)

In summary, Kanner offered the following "considerations":

(1) Early infantile autism is a well-defined syndrome which an experienced observer has little difficulty in recognizing in the course of the first two years of the life of the patient.

(2) The basic nature of its manifestations is so intimately related to the basic nature of childhood schizophrenia as to be indistinguishable from it, especially from the cases with insidious onset.

(3) Nevertheless, one can hardly speak of an insidious onset of early infantile autism . . . there may be a slow onset of the ability to recognize the child's behavior for what it represents but the condition as such is unquestionably there.

(4) Early infantile autism may therefore be looked upon as the earliest possible manifestation of childhood schizophrenia. As such, because of the age at the time of the withdrawal, it presents a clinical picture which has certain characteristics of its own, both at the start and in the course of later development. I have tried to do justice to this by including the discussion of early infantile autism in the schizophrenia chapter of the rewritten edition of my textbook of Child Psychiatry (published in 1948), at the same time acknowledging its special features by dealing with it under a special subheading.

(5) I do not believe that there is any likelihood that early infantile autism will at any future time have to be separated from the schizophrenias, as was the case with Heller's disease.

(6) Nosologically, therefore, the great importance of the group which I have described as early infantile autism lies in the correction of the impression that a comparatively normal period of adjustment must precede the development of schizophrenia. . . . It also confirms the observation, made of late by many authors, that childhood schizophrenia is not so rare as was believed as recently as twenty years ago. (pp. 419–420)

Kanner experienced major difficulties as a result of a selection bias that he neither suspected nor anticipated. The families of his autistic population were, by his own description, "rather successful in their chosen careers." Family histories of "hospitalized" psychosis were practically nonexistent among the first- and second-degree relatives of his cohort, and most of his patients were drawn from the upper-middle class. The parents of autistic children were described as "emotionally frigid" individuals for whom "the child is essentially the object of an interesting experiment and can be put aside when he is not needed for this purpose." He did recognize that "not one of the parents has displayed any really creative abilities" and that they were "essentially conservative repeaters of that which they have been taught."

Toward the end of this paper Kanner acknowledged that the parents had been able to rear other "normal" children, so that he himself wondered if the personalities of the parents might be a milder expression of the same basic defect so dramatically expressed in the children (A31).

Lauretta Bender's work on childhood schizophrenia began in 1935; her first paper on the subject appeared in 1941–1942, and the classic and most-quoted paper appeared in 1947. As has been done with Despert and with Kanner, I shall use one of Bender's later papers (Bender, Freedman, Grugett, & Helme, 1952) to discuss her monumental work. She reports:

> As of Jan. 1, 1952, there are on file over 600 cases of Childhood Schizophrenia diagnosed since 1935. . . . Our present formulation is that Childhood Schizophrenia is a developmental lag at the embryological level, characterized by embryonic plasticity of the biological processes from which subsequent behavior evolves by maturation. The biological areas are best defined according to Gesell's concepts described in "The Embryology of Behavior," namely, homeostatic mechanisms, tonic-neck-reflex motor patterning, muscular tone, respiratory patterns, and waking and sleeping with changing states of consciousness. In other words, Childhood Schizophrenia displays developmental lags at the embryological level in these biological areas and the disturbed functioning is characterized by embryonic plasticity . . . a plastic type of immature behavior disorder in these areas of functioning, as the primary symptomatology. Anxiety and neurotic defense mechanisms are secondary and tertiary symptoms. (Bender et al., 1952, p. 67)

In this 1952 paper Bender et al. tested the validity of her diagnostic criteria for diagnosing childhood schizophrenia by comparing the frequency with which these criteria were observed in 30 schizophrenic children with their prevalence in 30 nonschizophrenic children, who had been "matched for sex (all boys), age, socioeconomic status and homes in which the children were brought up." Bender placed her criteria in six categories:

1. Vasovegetative or homeostatic functions;
2. Motor behavior;
3. Body-image and self-world perception;
4. Fantasy productions and reality testing;
5. Perception of and response to interpersonal relations;
6. Manifest anxiety and neurotic symptoms. (p. 69)

Bender *et al.* reported: "When the criteria appeared most closely concerned with the inner biological core the most marked difference between the schizophrenics and non-schizophrenics appeared." Specifically, significant differences between the schizophrenic and nonschizophrenic children were reported to have occurred in:

> "vascular, homeostatic abnormality (includes response to pain, noise, temperature, and tactile stimuli); . . . irregularity in eating–sleeping pattern; . . . motor hypoactivity and hypervariation; . . . whirling, cohesiveness; . . . [and] voice, speech abnormality" (1952, chart II, p. 71).

In another 1952 paper, Bender and Freedman described the first 3 years of life of eight schizophrenic children, with material drawn from the baby books kept by the children's parents.* Many of their findings are echoed in Chapters 2 through 4 of this book, for example, the tendency of schizophrenic infants to gag on new foods and to have difficulty with solids, the failure of the schizophrenic baby to "respond with the reserve of muscle tone" when picked up, the fear of moving objects, the "extremely flexible hands and feet," the hypotonicity, the lack of complex gross motor development, the cessation of normal babbling, the lethargy, the lack of spontaneous activity, the peculiar attachment to hard transitional objects, the extreme fearfulness, the development of compulsive, destructive play, the abnormal gait, the fluctuating state of arousal, and the sleep disturbances.

During the same year that Kanner wrote his historic paper, Lourie, Pacella, and Piotrowski (1943) published the first follow-up study of 20 youngsters who, prior to age 12, had been diagnosed as suffering from childhood schizophrenia. The youngsters were all seen at the New York State Psychiatric Institute and were diagnosed using Potter's six

---

*Other publications have described in some details the first years of life of children who developed schizophrenia: (1) M. Tramer's "Diary of a Psychotic Child" (1941–1942); (2) Darr and Worden's 1951 case report of a 28-year-old who had suffered from an infantile autistic disorder; (3) two case histories included in a special issue of *Nervous Child* on childhood schizophrenia in 1952 (Harms, 1952); (4) and a case report of a 3-year-old described by Elizabeth Langer in the same special issue (Langer, 1952).

criteria. All of the subjects had been "neurologically negative at the time of the original study" and each had been regarded as a "deterioration from previously higher levels of adjustment." Four to 11 years (the average being 8 years) had elapsed from the time of "extended critical survey on the ward":

> The present adjustment levels of our series of children seemed to be classifiable into three main groups, as follows: I. Apparently normal adjustment in the community, educationally and socially (4 cases). II. Fair to borderline adjustments in the community—this includes fair or good educational adjustment with poor social adjustment (5 cases). III. Low grade adjustments which may be further subdivided into three types (usually in institutions): (a) Typical adult schizophrenic reaction types (3 cases). (b) Maintaining the same level as when originally seen, or further deteriorated (5 cases). (c) Reactions as in "b" but in which an organic basis has been established (3 cases). (Lourie et al., 1943, p. 543)

Childhood Schizophrenia or Mental Retardation?

From 1948 to 1954, a number of papers appeared in the literature that examined the relationship between childhood schizophrenia and mental retardation (Angus, 1948; Bergman, Waller, & Marchand, 1951; O'Gorman, 1954; Richards, 1951).

In 1948, Leslie Angus, mindful of Potter's admonition to look for schizophrenia among patients in institutions for mental deficiency, reported the following incidence: Of 150 consecutive admissions to Devereux over a period of 13 months—and despite a policy that grossly psychotic children could not be admitted—"there were 43 cases or about 28% of the admissions which could be diagnosed as schizophrenic, varying in degree from unquestionable psychoses to less well defined cases" (p. 227). Angus divided his cases into two groups:

> The larger group of 34 is composed of older children and presents, in general, the classical picture of schizophrenia recorded in the textbooks of psychiatry. . . . The second group which is smaller (9 cases of which 4 were considered established and 5 early, but not confirmed) consists of the schizophrenias of childhood. (p. 228)

In arriving at a diagnosis of childhood schizophrenia, Angus used the criteria of Potter, which require that there be a thought disturbance, and he admitted that had "we been a little more elastic in our criteria we should have included another 4 or possibly 5 cases." The detailed case descriptions included in this paper lend strong support to the author's diagnosis. Angus concludes: "There is a great deal more to be learned about such early conditions and much that can be learned in special schools if we will but devote the time and thought to the problem" (p. 237).

By far the most comprehensive paper on this subject was published by B. W. Richards in 1951. Richards sought to determine how many childhood schizophrenics were confined to his institution and to ascertain the following: "(1) Relationship of age of onset to resulting mental grade and degree of dementia. (2) Relationship of intensity of disease process to form of symptoms. . . . (3) Relationship of age of onset to form of symptoms" (p. 291).

Richards believed that it was important to distinguish between "mental grade" and "dementia" (A32). He divided his cases into those in which "Absence of Original Defect Appears to Be Certain" and those in which it is "Not Certain that Schizophrenia Is Present without Original Defect." His comments on the dilemma of determining whether the mental defect is primary or not are thoughtful (A33).

Richards reached a number of important conclusions regarding the relative importance of "age of onset" (A34) and "severity of illness" (A35). He also attributed some prognostic significance to "body build" (A36). He summarized his conclusions by attempting to classify the forms of schizophrenia that he had encountered among the mentally defective (reminding his readers that even the "mildest" of these cases has been institutionalized):

(1) Mild. Insidious onset. Schizophrenia simplex is the typical form. Simple paranoid tendencies may develop later and obsessive ruminative thought content. Fairly good preservation of personality.

(2) Moderate. Hebephrenic features quite common often combined with catatonic features. Symptoms in verbal and psy-

chomotor spheres. Difficult or impossible to converse with. Sometimes able to read and write.

(3) Severe. Psychomotility disorder, hyperkinesia. Idiocy. No speech. Incontinence. . . . When symptoms are apparent in the ideational sphere only, the prognosis is least gloomy, the mental level may be within normal limits and social contact retained. (1951, p. 306)

With regard to "propfschizophrenia," schizophrenia engrafted upon mental retardation, Richards maintained:

The frequency with which it is reported would be much diminished by careful histories and mental testing, where possible. A number of cases diagnosed as propfschizophrenia might be shown either to have been normal in infancy or else still to be normal on mental tests. (p. 309)

In conclusion Richards stated:

Patients with childhood schizophrenia are quite often disposed of to mental deficiency institutions. They are usually not diagnosed as such or seen by psychiatrists before admission. Most often they present as behavior problems to the parents or educational problems to the local authorities, and are diagnosed as mentally defective without further qualification. (p. 310)

In yet another study of the relationship between childhood schizophrenia and mental deficiency, Bergman *et al.* (1951) made the observation that:

one is reluctant to call children psychotic, evidently because of the gravity of such a designation and—what is more likely—because of the lack of facilities for the treatment of psychotic children. . . . The institutional system is geared to adult psychotics and mentally defective children. (p. 295)

Bergman *et al.* estimated that 15% of the admissions to Newark State School were schizophrenic. Like Richards, they divided their cases into three categories:

Nuclear schizophrenic reactions erroneously diagnosed as mental deficiency . . . cases of oligophrenia with superimposed schizophrenic patterns . . . and cases in which the writers were unable to discern any distinct schizophrenic patterns on Rorschach and psychological tests, to account for the unusual behavior. (p. 311)

In the case histories following this categorization, the authors described a case that met Heller's descriptions, a case that met Kanner's descriptions, and a paranoid schizophrenic child, as well as a number of cases of "reactive schizophrenia." The authors acknowledged this heterogeneity by stating that "in the general population at Newark State School, one notes a wide range of schizophrenic symptomatology."

In a 1954 paper Gerald O'Gorman reported on his efforts to determine the percentage of schizophrenic individuals who were inmates of (1) a villa for "low-grade female defectives" and (2) "a villa for mentally defective boys under 14 years." In the female villa, O'Gorman reported that: "29 percent of the patients were regarded as psychotic. In each case the clinical picture was indistinguishable from that of deteriorated schizophrenia" (p. 935).

In the boys' villa six of 43 children (14%) were identified as "psychotic, without history of epilepsy or signs of organic cerebral disease," and 14 more boys were identified as "insufficiently investigated" (p. 936). An interesting observation made by O'Gorman was that the ward for "babies" contained no psychotics. He speculated on this absence of cases in children younger than 5 years old:

> "Suppose juvenile schizophrenia were really a cause rather than a sequela of mental deficiency, then this absence of cases under 5 would be expected, since the disease would have to progress considerably before the child would be considered sufficiently retarded to be diagnosed as mentally defective. (p. 936)

O'Gorman concluded that there is evidence of the existence of both a "catatonic psychosis of idiocy" and a "hebephrenic psychosis of imbecility." He wondered if there might be, to complete the picture, a "simple schizophrenic psychosis of feeblemindedness":

> Schizophrenia beginning in childhood is a cause of mental deficiency. If severe and associated with much deterioration it causes imbecility or idiocy. If simple (or mild or early), it tends to produce feeblemindedness. (p. 936)

Finally, in a paper that described in much detail the "Application of Psychological Tests and Methods of Schizophrenia in Children," Helen Mehr (1952) acknowledged that:

With regard to Feeblemindedness, during the author's experience as a clinical psychologist, she has been impressed with the large number of children referred as school problems whose Rorschach records seemed to have the type of withdrawal mechanisms and inefficient mental functioning associated with the schizoid type of personality. Moreover many of the children who were referred for testing as possible candidates for mentally retarded classes (i.e. classes for children with I.Q.'s below 75) showed typical signs of disordered mental functioning, bizarre fantasy and flat affect associated with schizophrenia. (p. 90)

The Pediatricians Comment

As the decade of the 1950s began, Harry Bakwin contributed several papers to the pediatric literature designed to familiarize pediatricians with the signs and symptoms of childhood mental illness (Bakwin, 1950a, 1950b, 1951). Bakwin was a strong advocate for "providing better diagnostic and educational facilities for the mentally handicapped." By 1950 he was warning pediatricians: "Schizophrenia may also cause sufficient withdrawal of the child to suggest severe mental retardation. Skillfull psychiatric study is necessary for accurate diagnosis of childhood psychoses" (1950a, p. 424).

Also in 1950, under the heading "Psychologic Aspects of Pediatrics" (1950b), Bakwin described childhood schizophrenia. He cited Bradley and Bender extensively, including a description of Bender's motor and vasovegetative signs. He also detailed many of the typical findings on psychometric examination. Bakwin urged pediatricians to "suspect the diagnosis of schizophrenia in every severely disturbed child": "In schizophrenia, as distinguished from simple mental retardation, development proceeds normally at first and then either slows down or deteriorates" (1950b, p. 423).

Finally, he advised that:

severe behavior disorders, accompanied by excessive anxiety, are sometimes distinguished with difficulty from schizophrenia. In such instances the children should be referred to an institution where they can receive prolonged psychiatric observation. (1950b, p. 423)

By 1951, in a short comment on pediatrics in general practice, Bakwin remarked that childhood schizophrenia was "coming to be recognized with increasing frequency."

However, Bakwin's warmth toward psychiatry and toward childhood schizophrenia was in sharp contrast to an article by Jeanne Smith published in *Archives of Pediatrics* in 1951. Smith took exception to all aspects of childhood schizophrenia, especially the biological methods of treatment which were in vogue in 1951. These treatments she identified as "new methods of psychiatric procedures . . . [they] include insulin and metrazol shock, electric shock and the latest method of somatic psychiatric treatment, prefrontal lobotomy" (p. 477).

Smith quoted extensively from Bender's descriptions of schizophrenia in childhood and concluded that "no child would be entirely safe from the diagnosis of schizophrenia." She dismissed Bender's descriptions of "plasticity" as a "self-contradictory syndrome" and persisted in interpreting everything that Bender said in the most concrete terms.

Smith used Bradley's reference to schizophrenia as a "way of life" as a means to demand whether one should treat a "way of life" with electric shocks. Despert was similarly misunderstood and dismissed. Even when Smith cited some of the retrospective studies of adult schizophrenia that revealed many signs of vulnerability in childhood, she clung to statements in the literature such as the following:

> There can be no doubt that some individuals with withdrawn personalities will become schizophrenic, but this is quite different from saying that all withdrawn types are potential schizophrenics. (Smith, 1951, p. 482, quoting Kemble)

Many of Smith's criticisms are made more painful by the fact that they all too accurately reveal the excesses to which psychiatry is prone:

> The purpose of prefrontal lobotomy for the schizophrenias occurring in childhood has been undertaken with a view to terminating the fantasy-life and reducing the expenditure of emotional energy upon the self. . . . (Smith, 1951, p. 484, quoting Freeman & Watts)

Smith concluded her paper with the admonition: *"Primum non nocere!* Above all do no harm."

1955–1988: WHERE ARE WE NOW?

What can be said of the more than 100 years of literature on schizophrenia in childhood that has just been reviewed? Are there trends? Are we wiser than we were 100 years ago? Are we any closer to definitive answers?

I have sampled the literature on schizophrenia in childhood in order to learn how five major questions have been considered:

1. What are the manifestations of schizophrenia in childhood?
2. What did maturity-onset schizophrenics look like as children?
3. Can we define vulnerability?
4. What is the relationship between schizophrenia in childhood and mental deficiency?
5. What happens to the children of diagnosed schizophrenics? What do these children look like?

All of these questions have continued to be pursued in the literature of the past 30 years. Psychotic children have been the object of intensive study, and several efforts have been made to classify them (Anthony, 1958; Creak, 1964; Fish, Shapiro, Campbell, & Wile, 1968; Goldfarb, 1961, 1967). In a sophisticated effort to address the "nature versus nurture" controversy, there have been rigorous studies of the "adopted-away" offspring of schizophrenic individuals (Rosenthal, Wender, Kety, *et al.*, 1968) The search for the nature of the "inherited vulnerability" has been ongoing (reviewed by Fish & Ritvo, 1979; and by Asarnow & Goldstein, 1986).

DSM-III and DSM-III-R

The American Psychiatric Association's most recent diagnostic manuals (DSM-III and its 1987 revision, DSM-III-R) have reverted to the system of diagnosis that obtained before Potter's 1933 paper: Children with schizophrenia are again being diagnosed using the same criteria as are applied to adults.

Psychiatry as a whole now places less emphasis on the "primary" symptoms of schizophrenia described by Bleuler and Kraepelin (which can fairly easily be observed in children) and more on the first-rank symptoms of Kurt Schneider, namely, hallucinations and delusions. Since almost all writers have agreed that the majority of children lack the mental sophistication to produce such symptoms before the age of 9 or 10, the diagnosis of schizophrenia in children has been made that much more difficult by this emphasis upon Schneiderian schizophrenia.

Similarly, we have moved far away from Kanner's definition of infantile autism. The traditional organic/functional dichotomy, to which Kanner adhered, has been abandoned and the definition of "autism" in DSM-III-R is now based upon the views of Lorna Wing (1985). Autism as now defined is firmly related to mental deficiency and, except in rare circumstances, bears little relationship to the schizophrenias.

The Question of "Vulnerability"

The exact nature of "vulnerability" has continued to be defined and redefined. During the past 30 years a vast literature on borderline personality disorders has developed. There is still no agreement on what might constitute the prodroma of schizophrenic disease and on who is vulnerable. Thought disorder in children continues to be wistfully dismissed as "developmental," despite Despert's study of the phantasy productions of normal children (Despert, 1940). In the interim, "vulnerable" children have received still another name: besides "schizoid" and "psychopathic," they may now also be referred to as showing Asperger's syndrome.

All this is despite the fact that Potter's children have been followed into adult life (Bennett & Klein, 1966), as have Bender's (Bender, 1970). These and other "follow-up" studies have been reviewed by Fish and Ritvo (1979). A diagnosis of schizophrenia has been confirmed, on follow-up, in the vast majority of Potter's and Bender's cases.

Finally, many retrospective studies of adult schizophrenics have been done, with the object of better understanding "vulnerability." The findings have tended to confirm those of Kasanin and Veo (1932). A comprehensive review of retrospective studies was published by Offord and Cross in 1969.

The "High-Risk" Studies

Some of the most exciting developments in the literature of the past 30 years have occurred in the "at-risk" literature. Barbara Fish succeeded Lauretta Bender at Bellevue and continued her extensive studies of schizophrenia in childhood. In addition, Fish began detailed studies of the offspring of schizophrenic mothers, which have confirmed that many of the disturbances in growth and vasovegetative functioning that had been reported to occur in childhood schizophrenia have also occurred in those children of schizophrenic mothers who would later develop recognizable schizophrenic disease. A detailed review of Fish's work can be found in the *American Handbook of Child Psychiatry* (Fish & Ritvo, 1979). Moreover, Marcus, (Marcus, Auerbach, Wilkonson, & Burack, 1981; Marcus, Hans, Mednick, Schulsinger, & Michelson, 1985), working with a cohort of Israeli families, have documented very similar disturbances in perceptual and sensorimotor functioning. A case history of a "high-risk" subject has recently been published by Fish in the *Journal of the American Academy of Child Psychiatry* (1986).

Childhood Schizophrenia or Mental Retardation?

Psychiatry's interest in the relationship between childhood schizophrenia and mental deficiency has waned in the last 30 years. I very much regret this, because I find that here in Manitoba, the descriptions published in the papers cited in this chapter (1948–1954) still hold true. Pediatricians here would understand Smith's 1951 article, and many would most heartily agree with her concrete interpretations. Much stigma surrounds the diagnosis of childhood schizophrenia, and pediatricians rarely make such a diagnosis. Most schizophrenic children go undetected until they "fall into mental retardation" in the manner described by Richards (1951), get into trouble with the law (a happening very frequently alluded to in the old literature: i.e., children are "perverted" once more), or become indisputably insane in the manner of adult schizophrenics. There is no conceivable way in which preventive ego reconstitutive work can be undertaken in the vast majority of cases. The children continue to reach us only after there has been major damage to their development.

I can only plead as I did in one of my own earlier publications: "Childhood Schizophrenia is present—we must account for it" (Cantor *et al.*, 1982).

CHAPTER TWO

THE PRESCHIZOPHRENIC INFANT AND TODDLER

Only rarely does the preschizophrenic infant give cause for concern to either the attentive parent or the conscientious physician. Most such infants sleep contentedly, remain alert and observant between feedings, respond to parental and familial attentions, are inclined to be attractive babies, and achieve the major motor milestones on time and in sequence. There is every reason to believe that, in at least half of those affected, the disease is not manifest at birth nor during the first year of life.

PREGNANCY, BIRTH, AND THE IMMEDIATE POSTNATAL PERIOD

Significant complications were reported to have occurred in seven of the 47 cases in whom we were able to obtain a detailed pre- and postnatal history.

These complications included five cases in which the expectant mother was hypertensive, two of whom developed preeclampsia. Two of these five births proceeded vaginally and without incident. In the other three cases the babies were delivered by cesarean section. Mother and child recovered uneventfully in two cases, but the third infant was premature and required a month in hospital to reach normal weight. He too developed perinatally without complications.

A sixth high-risk case involved a pregnancy in which no weight gain was recorded during the ninth month. The mother was hospitalized during the final month and induced at term, and the baby was born vaginally, weighing 7 lb, 8 oz.

The seventh high-risk birth involved a placenta previa that apparently was not diagnosed prior to delivery. A 4 lb, 3 oz baby was delivered vaginally 6 weeks prematurely and spent 2 weeks postnatally in the intensive care nursery. The baby was noted to be cyanotic at birth but recovered quickly and without complications.

Minor complications were reported to have occurred in nine more of our 47 cases. Meconium staining and a delay in breathing were noted at one birth (after an 18-hour labor), three babies were reported to have suffered only a "delay in breathing," two babies were born with the cord wrapped around the neck, one child was "held back until the doctor came," one child was delivered by cesarean section after 36 hours of nonprogressive labor, and one mother was transported from a rural to a city hospital after 32 hours of nonprogressive labor. Only the latter baby (induced intravenously and delivered vaginally) experienced any perinatal difficulties, requiring several days in the intensive care nursery to stabilize. None of the other births caused concern at the time they occurred. All were regarded as noteworthy only in retrospect.

FEEDING BEHAVIOR OF THE PRESCHIZOPHRENIC CHILD

Major feeding disturbances were relatively rare in the group of 29 preschizophrenic infants on whom we have detailed developmental histories. In a few cases, moderate to severe motor dysfunction was present from birth. Six of our 29 cases were reported to have "poor suck," although the problem was severe in only one child, who "fell asleep at the breast or with a bottle." This baby was hospitalized at 1 month of age for "failure to thrive." A nursing report documented that it took 3 hours to administer 3 oz of formula!

Despite the infrequent occurrence of major feeding disturbances in preschizophrenic infants, the potential centrality of feeding to the mother–infant relationship is likely to bring to physician attention any difficulty that does occur. Such dysfunction should alert the attending physician to begin to carefully document motor development and to arrange to examine the affected infant at frequent intervals (monthly would be ideal; at least bimonthly is recommended).

SLEEPING BEHAVIOR OF THE PRESCHIZOPHRENIC CHILD

Disturbances in the arousal state, during both the waking and the sleep cycle, are often the first "symptom" to cause parental concern. Three preschizophrenic infants (of our 29 index cases) were reported to "sleep almost constantly" during the first few months, yet by the age of 6 months, two of these three infants "refused to sleep at all." Ten of the 29 index cases were reported to be "very light sleepers" during the first year of life, requiring that everyone "tiptoe around" practically from birth. Five of these 10 light sleepers were irritable during the waking state as well. Nine of these 10 light sleepers developed significant sleep disturbances as they matured (during the second or the third year of life).

Severe nightmares were described in three of our 29 index cases during the first 2 years of life. In two cases the mother described holding the screaming infant in her arms and being unable to wake or make conscious contact with the infant. One of the two mothers did note that on several occasions the baby woke spontaneously from the nightmare, vomited, and then fall back asleep, all without showing any signs of recognition of the mother who was holding him in her arms. This baby was seen by neurology staff and investigated for a possible "sleep disorder or generalized seizure disorder." The examining neurologists found "no identifiable neurological disorder at this time—baby to return for follow-up examination in 6 months." The nightmares abated, and the mother did not return.

By the second or the third year of life serious sleep disturbances were beginning to be noted and reported by most of the parents of our preschizophrenic toddlers. Some type of sleep disturbance occurred in 21 of our 29 index patients. "Difficulty falling asleep" ("he just can't seem to relax") was by far the most common problem, having been reported to occur in 18 of our 29 index patients by the age of 36 months (including the child whose nightmares have been described). In four of the 29 toddlers, difficulty falling asleep and staying asleep, and early morning awakening were all described; in a further nine children difficulty falling asleep and staying asleep were described; in six children difficulty falling asleep was the only identified problem; and in one child early morning awakening was the only problem (the 21st sleep-disturbed child was a child who slept excessively during the first few months but showed no evidence of sleep disturbance as he matured). Most parents did seek physician help and advice with the child's sleep disturbance; little success was reported, although one physician over-reacted and certified a schizophrenic child as mentally retarded in order to admit him to a provincial institution for a few months and allow his single parent to "catch up on her sleep."

The potential danger to a sleep-disturbed toddler posed by a sleeping household should be cause for physician concern. In carefully selected cases, physician response to parental complaints of a sleepless child is mandatory. Small doses of diphenhydramine (25 mg) are recommended for 2- to 5-year-olds, who not only waken frequently but also roam the house fearlessly and unattended once awake. Both sleep behavior and the understanding of potential danger tend to improve as the child matures; in fact, schizophrenic children often become cautious and fearful as their awareness of an alien world increases.

Difficulty falling asleep and staying asleep may remain recurring problems for some schizophrenic children throughout their developing years. As soon as they are old enough to understand (usually by age 5 or 6) it is therefore advisable to teach schizophrenic children to remain quietly in bed with a favorite book or toy (or sometimes soothing music) until they fall back asleep.

EARLY MOTOR DEVELOPMENT

Most preschizophrenic children achieve the early motor milestones on time and with little obvious effort. Two of our 29 children were even reported to be precocious in their motor development. Only five of our 29 children did not walk prior to 18 months. These five children were all noted by their parents to be lethargic ("lazy") or fearful, or both. In no case was the attending physician concerned about neurological development.

A very few preschizophrenic infants were noted to have severe motor abnormalities even during the first year of life. One of our 29 index patients required eye-patching for strabismus by 5 weeks of age. Six of our 29 patients encountered significant difficulty with chewing solid food. Three of the index 29 were fitted with special splints in infancy or special shoes as soon as they began to walk.

More often, significant motor dysfunction was not noted until complex motor activities were attempted by the affected child. Difficulty mastering stairs was experienced by seven of the 29 children. Nine of the 29 children were noted by physicians to toe walk or "waddle" abnormally by 3–4 years of age.

Family photographs of preschizophrenic children would suggest that the motor development of most is normal during the first year of life. Sometime during the second year of life (my own experience would suggest at 18–24 months) a child who had hitherto sat independently begins to constantly lean against his caretakers or a seat back, or on a table (Figure 1). It would appear that this "leaning" marks the onset of the hypotonia that has been a positive finding on physical examination in more than 90% of schizophrenic children (see Chapter 5).

EARLY SOCIAL DEVELOPMENT

The majority of preschizophrenic infants and toddlers in our group of 29 cases were reported to be smiling, responsive babies, at least during the first year of life (Figure 2). Most of these infants anticipated and liked being picked up (18 of 29 cases), responded joyfully to crib toys (20 of 29 cases), were curious infants (23 of 29 cases), babbled both spontaneously (20 of 29 cases) and in response to caretaker verbal stimulation (19 of 29 cases), and preferred company to being left alone (19 of 29 cases).

There were, of course, infants who were observed to be socially deviant even during the first year of life. Four of our 29 families reported that although their preschizophrenic infant appeared to enjoy being picked up, the baby did not

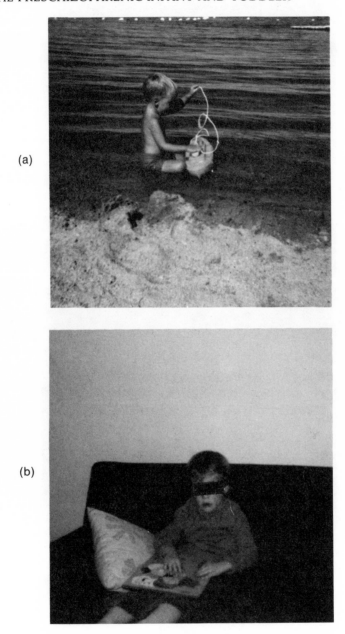

Figure 1
(a) A schizophrenic child at age 18 months (sitting erect and playing in the water). (b) The same child at age 3 years (leaning against the couchback doing a puzzle).

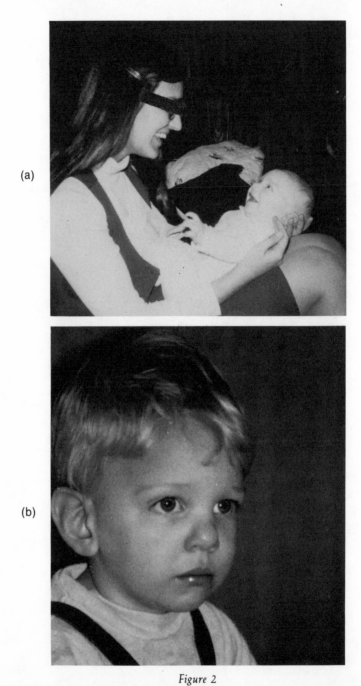

Figure 2
(a) A symptom-free preschizophrenic infant at age 3 months, happily interacting with his mother. (b) The same child at age 2 wearing the worried look
so characteristic of preschizophrenic toddlers.

anticipate (expectantly raise his/her arms) such pickup. A further six parents reported that even in infancy their child had either been indifferent to or openly resistant to parental handling, some babies having responded to cuddling by visably stiffening. Ten of our 29 index cases had seemed content to be left alone, even in infancy, a few crying irritably when obliged to interact with caretaking adults. The occasional infant (1 of our 29 cases) had latched on to a single caretaker and refused to be fed or cared for by anyone else.

Many of our preschizophrenic infants and toddlers had embraced a transitional object, such as a teddy bear or a favorite blanket (14 of our 29 cases). A few infants had chosen odd, hard objects, (such as cars, trucks, pot lids, etc.) to take to bed with them. In some cases worried parents had tried to modify the child's behavior by replacing the hard object with a softer stuffed animal. In all such cases (five of our 29 cases) the child had perseverated and the adult had been obliged to allow the child to keep the preferred hard object.

As the preschizophrenic children described here entered the second and the third year of life, deviant social behavior became more obvious. Nine of our index cases were observed to ignore peers, quickly moving to a safe distance when in the presence of other infants and toddlers. Six of the 29 children responded to the presence of peers by insisting on dominating the interaction (i.e., being very "bossy"), and three of the 29 children would interact with only one child at a time, hastily retreating in the presence of a larger group of children. Eight of the 29 children were observed to prefer adults to children, constantly seeking the attention of adults rather than interacting appropriately with their peers.

Nursery and day care reports on preschizophrenic children were peppered with comments on inappropriate interactions: "He lives in a world of his own." "He seems not to comprehend the things that other children do."

- "It is difficult to get and hold his attention."
- "He really only learns when I give him individual attention."
- "He behaves so strangely with other children: He either walks right up to them in the strangest way or he won't go near them at all."

EARLY COGNITIVE DEVELOPMENT

During the first year of life 25 of our 29 index cases were believed by their families to be "interested in their environment." Most also remarked that their child was curious (23 of 29) and became more curious as he or she matured. Two of our 29 index families described a baby who began life curious, babbling, and responsive, and who "fell silent and lost interest in everything at about 1 year of age." One mother noted that as her child matured, he remained curious but became more and more fearful and less and less willing to explore. Two parents reported that their child began to walk, fell a few times, and then refused to try again.

Much of the preschooler's early cognitive development depends upon the child's being able to observe, to imitate, to explore, to experiment (using a rapidly maturing sensorimotor system), to learn from experience, and to generalize that which is learned to other, similar situations or occurrences (in Piagetian terms, the infant and toddler must be able to "assimilate" and to "accommodate"). Given the amount of material to be mastered during the first 5 years of life, the infant and child is, not surprisingly, externally directed, more often scanning and observing large amounts of data than focusing on and mastering the minutiae. The schizophrenic preschooler's attention unfortunately appears to be divided between the internal and the external. This child tends to be a "trivialogist," preoccupied with minute details while failing to observe the whole (Cantor, 1982; Norman, 1954).

The early cognitive development of preschizophrenic children can perhaps best be understood by considering in some detail the ways in which these children seem to gather and process information.

Ability to Observe and Imitate

Preschizophrenic children are handicapped in several ways in their ability to observe and imitate:

1. 20% of schizophrenic children have evidence of clinically significant external eye muscle dysfunction (strabismus; see Chapter 5, Table 14).

2. A shortened attention span was severe enough in almost all of our 29 index cases to be observed and reported by both parent and nursery school teacher.

3. Many of our preschizophrenic children appeared to respond as readily to internal stimuli as to the external environment (withdrawal, preoccupation; see Chapter 4, Table 13).

4. The observations of schizophrenic preschoolers tended to be fragmented (fragmented thought; see Chapter 5, Figure 7).

5. The sensory system of schizophrenic children was observed to be hyperaroused and nonselective; that is, a schizophrenic child is as likely to heed the sound of footsteps in the hallway as the sound of the teacher's voice within the classroom (hyperacusis; see Chapter 5, Figure7). Perhaps as a defense against overstimulation, preschizophrenic children tend to try to avoid sensory stimulation (e.g., they may be withdrawn, rather than good observers).

6. Preschizophrenic children are frequently observed to be lethargic and hypoaroused, perhaps as a result of, or as yet another manifestation of the sleep disturbance already described.

Ability to Explore and Experiment

Several factors combine to inhibit the preschizophrenic child's ability to explore and experiment:

1. Deficits in both gross and fine motor functioning prevent active exploration (hypotonia, decreased muscle power, decreased muscle mass; see Chapter 5, Figure 4).

2. Preschizophrenic children are fearful (anxiety; see Chapter 5, Figure 7).

3. By the third year of life perseverative behavior was interfering with the child's ability to learn by doing in 14 of our 29 cases.

4. The young child's intuitive ability to use toys as object representations and to use fantasy-play as a means of

projecting real-life situations onto toys and achieving a sense of mastery, is not available to preschizophrenic children. Fewer than 25% of our index cases showed any ability to fantasy-play appropriately, by far the majority of the children using toys perseveratively and idiosyncratically (see Chapter 5).

Ability to Learn from Experience and to Generalize from What Is Learned

Since the child experiences the world by observing, imitating, exploring, and experimenting, it is evident from the foregoing discussion that the ability of preschizophrenic children to learn from experience is severely limited. In fact, as the nursery teacher quoted previously remarked, these children learn very little spontaneously. In a safe environment they can be observed to engage in very repetitive sensorimotor play; for example, they will roll toy vehicles back and forth by the hour, pile building blocks endlessly, constantly take apart and reassemble building toys, play by the hour with toys that have movable parts, or line up everything they can find in orderly rows. Some children refuse to play with anything other than number or alphabet games. These they will sequence over and over again. A few children become very gifted at assembling jigsaw puzzles. The occasional child who does engage in fantasy-play can usually be overheard acting out exactly what he or she has seen on television (a form of delayed echolalia) rather than projecting any real-life situations onto his or her toys.

The special cognitive deficits of the preschizophrenic child are usually revealed all too clearly by the child's lack of spontaneous speech (poverty of speech and poverty of content of speech; see Chapter 5, Figure 12), and by the relative rarity with which preschizophrenic children ask information-seeking questions. When such children reached elementary school without being detected, conscientious teachers often requested a psychological assessment on the basis of the child being "too quiet" and "hardly even knowing he's there." The questions that preschizophrenic children did ask more often sought reassurance ("Can we go home now?") than information.

SPECIAL DEVELOPMENTAL CONCERNS

Toilet Training

Just over half of the 29 index cases were toilet trained at home with little difficulty. Six of the 29 children were trained by the staff of the special-needs programs in which they were enrolled. Five more were finally trained at home by 6 years of age. Intermittent enuresis, both by day and by night, was frequently observed, especially in the preschizophrenic or the schizophrenic child who was easily agitated or overstimulated.

I would like to emphasize here that, due to the many signs of cholinergic dysfunction observed in schizophrenic children (Cantor *et al.*, 1980, 1981, 1982), anticholinergic medication for enuresis (e.g., imipramine) is contraindicated. The author has seen at least one preschizophrenic 6-year-old in whom a schizophreniform psychosis was precipitated by the administration of imipramine for nocturnal enuresis.

Autonomic Instability

Seventeen of our 29 index cases were reported to have suffered high fevers during the second to the fifth year of life. Some parents reported that their children suffered fevers during relatively minor infectious episodes, such as upper respiratory infections (URIs) and uncomplicated middle ear infections, as well as fevers related to teething or to exposure to the sun, and sometimes for no reason that either the parent or the child's physician could identify. Most of the children had to be bathed to bring the fever down. None of these children suffered febrile seizures, although one boy in the larger group of 47 youngsters on whom we have detailed histories did require phenobarb for febrile convulsions until 6 years of age.

Unusual Behaviors and Fears

Most of our 29 index cases displayed some form of "unusual" behavior by the age of 3 years (18 of 29). Rocking (one child wore out two rocking chairs) and motor agitation were the most common behaviors reported (occurring in eight of the 29 children), followed by head banging (six of the 29);

perseverative behaviors such as opening and closing telephone booth doors, twirling objects, or compulsively turning lights on and off (six of 29 cases); smelling, mouthing, or touching everything (six of 29 cases); biting and scratching (three of 29 cases); hand flapping (two of 29 cases); and lack of attention to danger (one of 29 cases).

Most preschizophrenic children (17 of 29 cases) began to react with fear and angry outbursts to loud noises by the second year of life. The lawn mower, the vacuum cleaner, airplanes, trucks, and thunderstorms—all were identified as sources of terror for preschizophrenic children. One child was so terrified of mosquitos that he refused to go outside for two seasons; another reacted in a similar manner to canker worms (calling the park in which he had first encountered the worms "scary park").

Moving toys, such as swings or rocking horses, were actively avoided by 14 of our 29 preschizophrenic toddlers. The children seemed to have a particular fear of going backward (as happens on a swing). It may be of some interest that three of the children who were constant rockers during the first year of life actively avoided moving toys during the next 4 years of their lives (it is tempting to speculate that both the excessive rocking during the first year of life and the later avoidance of movement reflect the same disturbance in the vestibular system, albeit at a different stage in the pathology).

Other common fears of preschizophrenic children included water (four of 29 cases), the dark (four of 29 cases), labels on clothes (three of 29 cases), hair cuts and hair washes (two of 29 cases), school (three of 29 cases), being touched (three of 29 cases), and strangers (4 of 29 cases). Although some of these fears are not in themselves "unusual," the intensity of the preschizophrenic child's reaction (which may include screaming, crying for hours, throwing objects, total withdrawal and muteness, etc.) usually persuades the child's family to give in and quickly separate the child from that which is feared, even if it inconveniences the rest of the family.

CHAPTER THREE

ABOUT NORMAL CHILDREN

In order to gain some insight into what distinguishes the schizo-phrenic child from a child who is developing more normally, the questionnaire (Appendix B) that had been completed by the parents of our study cohort was distributed to the parents of 64 age-matched controls, 40 males and 24 females.*

Since our patient group contained too few females for meaningful statistical analysis, we compared the question-naires of the 40 control males with the questionnaires of the 27 males in our study cohort. For the sake of completeness the tables presented in this chapter do also provide all the data gathered on the 24 normal females, and the control females have been compared with the control males in an effort to determine what developmental differences, if any, might exist between the two sexes. (All statistically significant differences between groups are provided as footnotes to Tables 2–12).

FAMILY HISTORY

Schizophrenia-spectrum disease was reported significantly more frequently among the first- and second-degree relatives of the preschizophrenic and schizophrenic children (some of the children were already manifesting the symptoms of

---

*The participating parents of control children selected themselves from among a large group of day care parents who were approached. Less than 50% of the day care parents approached actually completed the question-naire. We were thus obliged to recognize that the questionnaire is too long and is, at least to some degree, "onerous." We therefore suspect that there was a tendency toward self-selection among those parents who had some concern about their own child's development (this suspicion was confirmed by the high prevalence rate of alcoholism and affective disorders within the control families; see Table 2).

schizophrenia at the time that the parents completed the questionnaire; others were mute and no diagnosis could yet be made) than in the families of the age-matched controls (Table 2). Surprisingly, alcoholism was significantly more prevalent in the families of the control children than the study children. Affective disorders were significantly more frequent in families of control males than control females. There was no significant difference between the families of the control and study groups when socioeconomic class was estimated using the scale of Hollingshead and Redlich (1953).

BIRTH AND PERINATAL COMPLICATIONS

There was no significant difference reported in the prevalence rate of birth complications between the control children and the study children (Table 3). Only one parameter, "perinatal instability," recorded any significant difference between the two groups, as within the study cohort one child was reported to have had "heart and stomach troubles," one child was "hypoglycemic," one child had a "cyanotic episode during the 1st feeding and had to be rushed away," one child was "cyanotic" and had to spend 5 days in the intensive care nursery (the child was a placenta previa baby), and one child was premature and needed time to "stabilize."

VEGETATIVE FUNCTIONING

The basic physiological functions such as "feeding," "sleeping," and "toilet training" revealed several important differences between the control children and the study children (Tables 4 and 5).

Feeding Difficulties

Although only 10% of control children experienced any difficulty with early feeding, more than 40% of the study children demonstrated some deviance in feeding behavior (Table 4). Feeding difficulties may well be the first sign of disordered functioning to attract the attention of the alert physician.

Table 2
Family history

Area of concern	Number of children affected			
	Control		Schizophrenic	
	Male (N = 40)	Female (N = 24)	Male (N = 27)	Female (N = 2)
Total with positive history	18 (45%)	10 (42%)	22 (81.5%)[a]	1 (50%)
Schizophrenia spectrum	0	1	14[b]	0
Affective disorders	11[d]	1	3	0
Alcoholism	13[c]	6	3	0
Epilepsy	3	1	2	0
"Nervous breakdown" or "mental illness"	1	2	4	1
Speech delay	2	0	2	0
Learning disability	0	0	0	1
Suicide	1	0	1	0
Phobias	0	1	1	0
Other neurological disorders	1	0	2	0
Mental retardation	2	0	3	0

Note. Data analysis was by chi square except where expected value was less than 5 and Fisher's exact test was used. Control males versus schizophrenic males: [a]$p < .01$; [b]$p = .000001$; [c]$p = .02$. Control males versus control females: [d]$p = .02$.

Table 3
Birth and perinatal complications

| | Number of children affected | | | |
| | Control | | Schizophrenic | |
Area of concern	Male (N = 40)	Female (N = 24)	Male (N = 27)	Female (N = 2)
Total with positive history	15 (37.5%)	11 (45.8%)	15 (55.5%)	1 (50%)
Elevated blood pressure	3	1	4	0
Prolonged labor	1	0	3	1
Unplanned cesarean	2	2	3	0
Cord around the neck	3	3	2	0
Delay in breathing	1	2	2	1
Meconium staining	2	1	1	0
Fetal distress	0	1	1	0
Gestational diabetes	2	0	0	0
Placenta previa	0	1	1	0
Neonatal jaundice	2	2	0	1
Perinatal instability	1	2	5[a]	0
Prematurity	0	3	2	0

Note. Data analysis was by chi square except where expected value was less than 5 and Fisher's exact test was used. Control males versus schizophrenic males: [a]$p = .035$.

Table 4
Feeding difficulties and sleep disturbance

	Number of children affected			
	Control		Schizophrenic	
Area of concern	Male (N = 40)	Female (N = 24)	Male (N = 27)	Female (N = 2)
Feeding difficulties				
Total with positive history	4 (10%)	3 (12.5%)	12 (44.4%)[a]	2 (100%)
Poor suck	0	2	4[b]	2
Resisting or regurgitating solids	4	1	9[c]	0
Odd food preference	0	0	5[d]	0
Sleep disturbance				
Total with positive history	12 (30%)	7 (29%)	19 (70.4%)	2 (100%)
Constant sleep at < 2 mo age	0	1	3	0
Difficulty falling asleep at > 36 mo	8	3	13[c]	1
Difficulty staying asleep at > 36 mo	4	3	10[e]	1
Early morning awakening at > 36 mo	3	2	6	0
Severe nightmares at < 24 mo	0	0	3	0

Note. Data analysis was by chi square except where expected value was less than 5 and Fisher's exact test was used. Control males versus schizophrenic males: [a] $p < .005$; [b] $p = .02$; [c] $p < .025$; [d] $p = .008$; [e] $p < .01$.

Table 5
Toilet training and high fever

| | Number of children affected | | | |
| | Control | | Schizophrenic | |
Area of concern	Male (N = 40)	Female (N = 24)	Male (N = 27)	Female (N = 2)
Toilet training				
Total who experienced difficulty	2 (5%)	0	11 (40.7%)[a]	1 (50%)
Witholding behavior	1	0	0	0
Resistance to training	2	0	5[b]	1
Unable to toilet train	0	0	6[c]	0
High fever				
Total with symptoms	21 (52.5%)	14 (58.3%)	16 (59.3%)	1 (50%)
Severe infections	2	2	1	0
Minor infections (URIs)	14	9	12	1
Middle ear infections	2	2	1	0
No known cause, heat induced	2	1	4	0
Febrile convulsions	4	1	1	0

Note. Data analysis was by chi square except where expected value was less than 5 and Fisher's exact test was used. Control males versus schizophrenic males: [a]$p < .0005$; [b]$p = .035$; [c]$p = .003$.

Sleep Disturbance

Sleep disturbance during the first 36 months of life was very common even among the control children (Table 4). By the fourth year of life, however, the sleep patterns of the control children were well established. Among children older than 36 months of age, a significantly greater number of schizophrenic children than control children continued to experience difficulty falling asleep and difficulty staying asleep.

Furthermore, although the numbers of children involved were too small to reach statistical significance, it should be noted that constant sleep during the first few months of life and severe nightmares at less than 2 years of age were reported to occur only in the study cohort.

Toilet Training

Only 5% of the control children were difficult to toilet train, although almost half of the study children presented some difficulty during training (Table 5). As noted in Chapter 1, at least six of the schizophrenic children were not toilet trained at home.

High Fever

Despite our clinical impression that high fevers were common phenomena in schizophrenic children and should be regarded as one of the symptoms of the disease, we were surprised to find that high fevers were common occurrences in normal preschoolers as well (Table 5). Although there was a trend for fevers due to "no known cause or heat" to occur more often in study children than in control children, there was no significant difference between the two groups.

ATYPICAL DEVELOPMENT

Early Social Interactions

There were no children within the normal cohort who, like the 10 infants described in Chapter 2, "preferred to be left alone" (Table 6). A lack of curiosity was only rarely reported to

Table 6
Atypical early social interactions

	Number of children affected			
	Control		Schizophrenic	
Area of concern	Male (N = 40)	Female (N = 24)	Male (N = 27)	Female (N = 2)
Total with some atypical social behavior	17 (42.5%)	6 (25%)	18 (66.7%)	2 (100%)
Disliked being picked up	3	0	5	0
Did not anticipate pickup	6[d]	0	8	2
Infant preferred to be alone	0	0	10[a]	0
No curiosity	2	1	6[b]	0
No soft objects cherished	9	3	10	1
Took hard objects to bed	1	0	5[c]	0
Limited social interactions	0	4[e]	3	0
No differentiation of major caretakers	11	2	7	0

Note. Data analysis was by chi square except where expected value was less than 5 and Fisher's exact test was used. Control males versus schizophrenic males: [a] $p = .00003$; [b] $p = .041$; [c] $p = .035$. Control males versus control females: [d] $p = .05$ (trend); [e] $p = .02$.

have occurred during the infancy of the control children, and only one of the control children was reported to take a hard object to bed with him.

Limited social interaction was more frequently observed in the control females (this was judged to be present if parents reported that their child related to just a few people and was somewhat reserved socially) than in the control males, whereas not anticipating pickup in early infancy was reported significantly more frequently in the control males than in the control females.

Play Behavior

Perseverative play was described in less than 10% of the control males and none of the control females. In contrast, almost 50% of the schizophrenic boys were observed by their parents to engage in stereotyped, repetitive play behavior (Table 7). A disinterest in toys was rarely observed to occur in the control children, and only one control child was reported to have ignored his crib toys.

Peer Behavior

Not surprisingly, it was in peer behavior that the most significant differences emerged between the schizophrenic children and the control children. Less than 10% of the control boys were reported to "prefer to play alone," compared with 1 of 3 of schizophrenic boys (Table 7). No control child was observed to ignore peers, whereas 8 of 27 schizophrenic boys did just that. Attempting to dominate peer interaction and becoming "hyper with peers" were behaviors observed only within the group of schizophrenic children.

Speech Development

Although 10% of the control males were reported to be mildly speech delayed ("no sentence development by age 36 months"; Table 8), significantly more schizophrenic children were seriously speech delayed. Schizophrenic children were significantly more likely to babble little in infancy, to be slow

Table 7
Atypical play and peer behavior

Area of concern	Number of children affected			
	Control		Schizophrenic	
	Male (N = 40)	Female (N = 24)	Male (N = 27)	Female (N = 2)
Play behavior				
Total with atypical play behavior	4 (10%)	2 (8.3%)	16 (59.3%)[a]	2 (100%)
Ignored crib toys	1	0	3	2
Disliked or disinterested in toys	0	1	3	1
Perseverative play	3	0	12[b]	1
Short attention span	0	1	0	0
Peer behavior				
Total with some unusual peer behavior	3 (7.5%)	3 (12.5%)	23 (85.2%)[c]	2 (100%)
Prefers to play alone	3	3	9[d]	1
Ignores peers	0	0	8[e]	1
Provokes fights with peers	0	0	1	0
Domineering or "hyper with peers"	0	0	7[f]	0
Plays with only one child at a time	0	2	3	0

Note. Data analysis was by chi square except where expected value was less than 5 and Fisher's exact test was used. Control males versus schizophrenic males: [a] $p < .0001$; [b] $p = .0005$, $p < .0003$; [c] $p = .0000001$, $p < .00001$; [d] $p = .009$, $p < .01$; [e] $p = .0003$; [f] $p = .001$.

Table 8
Atypical speech development

Area of concern	Number of children affected			
	Control		Schizophrenic	
	Male (N = 40)	Female (N = 24)	Male (N = 27)	Female (N = 2)
Total with atypical speech development	13 (32.5%)	6 (25%)	22 (81.5%)[a]	2 (100%)
Little early babble	1	0	8[b]	1
Slow to imitate parental vocalization	4	0	10[c]	0
No sentence development by 36 mo	4	1	22[d]	0
Reverse pronouns	6	2	5	0
Makes up words	5	5	9[c]	2
Severe dysarthria	1	0	1	0

Note. Data analysis was by chi square except where expected value was less than 5 and Fisher's exact test was used. Control males versus schizophrenic males: [a]$p < .0005$; [b]$p = .0022$; [c]$p < .05$; [d]$p < .0001$.

to imitate parental vocalization, and to fail to speak in sentences by 36 months of age. They were also more likely to "make up words" that were incomprehensible to the parent.

Motor Development

A surprising 10% of control males experienced some difficulty with mastering stairs (children who still could not ascend and descend stairs sequentially by 36 months of age). Nevertheless, significantly more schizophrenic children experienced a major motor milestone delay (Table 9), and an abnormal gait was observed in only 1 of the 40 control boys compared with 1 of 3 of the schizophrenic boys.

Motor Mannerisms

Almost half of the schizophrenic males were reported to engage in some type of repetitive motor behavior, compared with only 22.5% of the control males (Table 9). Many different types of behavior were seen, although rocking and head banging were the most prevalent.

IDIOSYNCRATIC BEHAVIORS

Unusual Fears

The control females were significantly more frequently reported to be fearful than the control males (Table 10). Schizophrenic males were reported to be significantly more fearful than control males, and even more fearful than control females. The fear of "moving toys and/or slides" best distinguished the schizophrenic children from both the control males and the control females. In addition, a fear of crowds or a fear of human contact was almost never reported to occur within the population of control children, but such fears occurred in more than 10% of schizophrenic children.

Unusual Behaviors

Repetitive "strange" behaviors were rarely reported to occur within the population of control children but were ob-

Table 9
Atypical motor development and mannerisms

Area of concern	Number of children affected			
	Control		Schizophrenic	
	Male ($N = 40$)	Female ($N = 24$)	Male ($N = 27$)	Female ($N = 2$)
Motor development				
Total with atypical motor development	4 (10%)	3 (12.5%)	16 (58.3%)[a]	2 (100%)
Hypotonia	0	0	1	1
Motor milestone delay	0	1	5[b]	0
Difficulty with stairs	4	1	6	1
Deformity requiring correction	0	2	3	0
Clumsiness	0	0	2	0
Abnormal gait	1	0	9[c]	0
Mannerisms				
Total with unusual motor mannerisms	9 (22.5%0	4 (16.7%)	13 (48.1%)[d]	0(0%)
Rocking	2	1	6	0
Head banging	2	0	5	0
Mouthing (after 18 mo)	4	1	4	0
Hand flapping	0	0	2	0
Repetitive jumping	0	1	1	0
Constant agitation	0	0	2	0
Clicking, snorting, breathholding	0	0	1	0
Self-abuse	1	1	0	0

Note. Data analysis was by chi square except where expected value was less than 5 and Fisher's exact test was used. Control males versus schizophrenic males: [a]$p < .0001$; [b]$p = .008$; [c]$p = .0001$; [d]$p < .01$.

Table 10
Unusual fears

| | Number of children affected | | | |
| | Control | | Schizophrenic | |
Area of concern	Male (N = 40)	Female (N = 24)	Male (N = 27)	Female (N = 2)
Total with unusual fear	12 (30%)	17 (70.8%)[d]	24 (88.9%)[a]	2 (100%)
Loud and/or sudden noises	8	12[e]	15[b]	2
Moving toys and/or slides	2	3	14[a]	0
Labels on clothes	0	3[f]	3	0
Monsters, "ghosts" (shadows)	3	1	3	0
Insects or worms	0	3[f]	2	0
Human contact	0	0	3	0
All humans except significant others	0	1	4[c]	0
Sparks of electricity	0	0	2	0
Crowds	0	0	2	0
Water	0	0	4[c]	0

Note. Data analysis was by chi square except where expected value was less than 5 and Fisher's exact test was used. Control males versus schizophrenic males: [a]$p < .0001$; [b]$p < .005$; [c]$p = .02$. Control males versus control females: [d]$p < .001$; [e]$p = .01$; [f]$p = .048$.

served in 40% of schizophrenic males.* Behaviors such as intermittent pacing, aimless wandering, smelling all objects, and perseverative tactile behaviors (e.g., compulsively touching everything) are all included in this category (Table 11).

Atypical Response to Frustration

In scoring this category, behaviors such as "sulking," "tantrumming," and so forth were regarded as normal, unless the sulking resulted in an extended period of social withdrawal or the tantrumming was reported to routinely result in the significant destruction of self or objects (these last two behaviors were scored as "self-abusive response" and "physically aggressive response"). A "paranoid response" was scored when it was reported that the child "hated to be laughed at" or "scowled and shook his fist at everyone."

No significant differences were noted between the schizophrenic children and the normal children in this category of behavior (Table 11), although there was certainly a trend for schizophrenic children to be more passive (no schizophrenic boy responded with a "physically aggressive" response, and "total withdrawal" was more frequently reported in the schizophrenic population). In fact, in my experience schizophrenic children tend to be very passive, avoiding frustration whenever possible ("It's too hard" is a frequently heard phrase in our early childhood classroom for schizophrenic children).

THE "VULNERABLE" CHILD

It was evident from the data that we had gathered (e.g., the family histories, the 10% of control children who were motor delayed and/or speech delayed, and the number of control children who displayed "unusual" behaviors, as well as deviant social, play, and peer-relationship behavior) that not all of the control children were "normal." Indeed, in any population of

*Author's note: In fact, such behaviors occurred in almost all schizophrenic children, but since the parents had often learned to "tune them out," they were documented in only 40% of the questionnaires.

Table 11
Unusual behavior and response to frustration

	Number of children affected			
	Control		Schizophrenic	
Area of concern	Male (N = 40)	Female (N = 24)	Male (N = 27)	Female (N = 2)
Unusual behavior				
Total with unusual behavior	2 (5%)	1 (4.2%)	11 (40.7%)[a]	1 (50%)
Unusual motor behaviors	0	0	4	0
Unusual sensory behaviors (excluding mouthing)	0	0	2	0
Fearlessness	0	0	1	0
Lining everything up	0	0	2	0
Insisting on eating alone, paranoid	0	0	2	0
Obsession with ideas or things	0	0	2	0
Hides when hurt	1	0	0	0
"Hyper," wears people out	1	1	1	0
Biting and/or scratching self and/or others	1	1	2	1
Response to frustration				
Total with atypical response to frustration	7 (17.5%)	4 (16.6%)	8 (29.6%)	2 (100%)
Self-abusive response	4	1	5	1
Physically aggressive response	3	2	0	1
Total withdrawal	0	1	3	0
Paranoid response	1	1	1	0
"Going stiff"	1	0	0	0

Note. Data analysis was by chi square except where expected value was less than 5 and Fisher's exact test was used. Control males versus schizophrenic males: [a]$p = .0004; p < .0005$.

Table 12
"Vulnerable" children

Case No. (sex)	FH	B & P	FD	SD	TT	HF	ASB	APB	UPB	ASD	AMD	UMM	UF	UB	ARF
12 (F)	−	−	−	−	−	+	−	+	−	−	−	−	+	+	−
17 (M)	+	+	−	−	−	+	+	+	−	+	−	+	+	+	+
23 (M)	−	+	+	+	−	−	−	−	−	−	−	−	+	+	+
30 (F)	+	−	−	−	−	−	+	−	+	−	−	−	+	+	−
35 (M)	+	+	+	+	−	−	+	−	+	+	−	−	+	−	−
42 (M)	+	−	−	+	+	+	−	+	+	−	+	+	+	−	−
47 (F)	−	+	−	−	−	−	+	−	+	−	−	−	+	−	−
60 (M)	+	−	−	−	−	+	+	−	+	−	−	−	+	−	−
61 (F)	−	+	+	+	−	+	+	−	+	+	−	−	+	−	+
% "vulnerable" controls affected (N = 9)	55.6	55.6	22.2	44.4	11.1	55.6	66.7^a	33.3^b	66.7^c	44.4	11.1	22.2	88.9^d	33.3^e	33.3
% nonvulnerable controls affected (N = 55)	41.8	38.2	9.1	27.3	1.8	54.5	30.9	3.6	0	27.3	10.9	20.0	38.2	0	14.5

Note. Data analysis was by Fisher's exact test. FH, family history; B & P, birth and perinatal complications; FD, feeding difficulties; SD, sleep disturbance; TT, toilet training; HF, high fever; ASB, atypical social behavior; APB, atypical play behavior; UPB, unusual peer behavior; ASD, atypical speech development; AMD, atypical motor development; UMM, unusual motor mannerisms; UF, unusual fears; UB, unusual behavior; ARF, atypical response to frustration. "Vulnerable" control males versus nonvulnerable control males: $^a p = .047$; $^b p = .032$; $^c p = .000001$; $^d p = .0058$; $^e p = .0020$.

73

"randomly selected" children, there should be a percentage of children who will mature into adult psychotics.

The data that we had gathered were analyzed using a "logist" analysis (the statistical techniques used have been described by Dillion & Goldstein, 1984, and Walker & Duncan, 1967) and the major findings were summarized as follows.

Only two items significantly predict group membership: unusual peer behavior ($p = .0001$) and unusual behaviors ($p = .043$). Although the latter significantly discriminated between the groups in and of itself, it did not add to our ability to correctly classify the subjects. Using both variables (where $0 =$ absence and $1 =$ presence):

Item 1	Item 2	Predicted probability of abnormality
0	0	.0497
0	1	.3876
1	0	.8331
1	1	.9837

There were no children within the control cohort who demonstrated abnormalities on both items—that is, abnormalities in both the category of unusual peer behavior (Table 7) and the category of unusual behavior (Table 11)—compared with 10 of 27 schizophrenic males who demonstrated such abnormalities. In reality, we have no reason to suspect that any of the control children should be said to be "abnormal" or to belong with the group of schizophrenic children.

There were, however, among the 64 control children, nine children who were positive for either Item 1 (unusual peer behavior) or Item 2 (unusual behavior). Table 12 presents a profile of these nine children. It is of interest that these nine children differed significantly (Table 12) from the other 55 control children in five areas of functioning: atypical social behavior, atypical play behavior, unusual peer behavior, unusual fears, and unusual behaviors. The areas of dysfunctioning identified are reminiscent of the descriptions of "vulnerable" children reported in the old literature (Childers, 1931; Conolly, 1861–1862; Courtney, 1911; Farnell, 1914). It seems probable, therefore, that we have identified a group of "vulnerable" children.

CHAPTER FOUR

IS THERE AN ONSET?

The diagnosis of schizophrenia in childhood depends upon the documentation of formal thought disorder (see Chapter 5). A definitive diagnosis therefore requires the child to have communicative speech that is sophisticated enough to reveal a disturbance in either thought content or thought process or both. Since the majority of childhood schizophrenics are speech delayed (19 of our 29 index cases were not talking when they first came to physician attention), the diagnosis of childhood schizophrenia cannot usually be made prior to the fifth or sixth year of life.

The question of when the disease actually begins remains an open one (probably awaiting future laboratory confirmation). It seems highly probable that the motor, affective, interpersonal, perceptual, and physiologic phenomena that have been observed and described in the preschizophrenic child (Chapter 2) are all manifestations of the schizophrenic syndrome. Certainly inappropriate affect, high anxiety, unusual behaviors and fears, social withdrawal and isolation, lethargy, sleep disturbance, and hyperacusis (a "breakdown in the sensory filter" is the descriptive phraseology employed in the adult psychiatric literature) are all symptoms that have long been recognized as associated with the much more prevalent postpubertal-onset schizophrenic syndrome. Only motor signs have rarely been mentioned in the literature on maturity-onset schizophrenia.

Most parents of schizophrenic children cannot pinpoint a time of onset. Many describe a growing feeling of apprehension, the beginning of which is "too far back to remember." Several parents of schizophrenic children have written eloquent descriptions of the affected child (see Introduction, this volume; D. Spungen, 1983; Wilson, 1968). Most parents began the narrative with the child's birth.

Half of our parents did believe the child was relatively symptom-free during the first year of life (see next section). At least one of these parents acknowledged, however, that even in the newborn nursery her baby's quietness excited staff comment. Other parents dated the child's difficulties to a traumatic event: "He fell and hit his head when he was 18 months old" (although there was no loss of consciousness at the time), or "He seemed to stop developing and to go backwards when his father and I separated." A few parents were quite convinced there was an onset but could not pinpoint a time or link the onset to anything definite.

Several of the parents admitted to having no concerns about the child, and even to having enjoyed parenting an undemanding child (the passive children who were identified by teachers). A few parents were resentful of the school, and of medical attention as well, believing strongly that there was nothing wrong with the child and that, in any case, maturation would bring a cure. Several of the symptom-free were included in this last group. Continuing parent denial at the time of initial consultation makes it difficult to accept the perceptions of all who maintained that their child was symptom-free during the first year of life. Nevertheless, a close look at our 29 cases did suggest that at least in some cases a period of normal development preceded the onset of childhood psychosis.

THE SYMPTOM-FREE INFANT

In 11 of our 29 cases no sign of childhood psychosis had been documented during the first year of life. In four more cases no sign other than light or easily arousable sleep had been reported. These 15 "symptom-free" children had anticipated and liked being picked up, enjoyed and responded to crib toys, babbled, imitated parental sounds prior to 1 year of age, had been interested in their environment, demonstrated curiosity, demonstrated no unusual behaviors or mannerisms, and in general appear to have given their parents little cause for concern during the first year of life (see Chapter 2, Figure 2). Even three of the four light sleepers, who had been described as irritable during the waking state, seem to have settled after the first few months, as the rest of the first year of life passed uneventfully.

The 15 symptom-free children were slower to present to physicians with developmental or behavioral complaints, as only 13% of symptom-free infants, compared with 43% of symptomatic infants, were seen in consultation by age 2. A further 27% of the symptom-free, compared with 43% of the symptomatic, presented to physicians during the third or fourth year of life. The majority of those who had been symptom-free during the first year of life were not seen by a child psychiatry specialist until 4 years of age or later (60% of the symptom-free compared with 14% of the symptomatic). It is of interest that in our cohort of 29 cases there were seven children with no history of speech delay. All seven of these children were counted among the 15 children who had been reported to be symptom-free during the first year of life.

A history of significant birth complications could not account for the earlier presentation of the symptomatic infants as 20% (3 of 15) of the symptom-free babies and 21% (3 of 14) of the symptomatic had such a history. Minor birth complications had been documented in an additional 13% (2 of 15) of the symptom-free babies and 21% (3 of 14) of the symptomatic babies.

PRESENTING COMPLAINTS

The presenting complaints of 47 schizophrenic children are outlined in Table 13. These 47 youngsters include the 30 cases on whom data have previously been published (Cantor et al., 1982) and the 29 cases discussed in some detail in Chapter 2 (10 of those 29 index cases were also a part of the group of 30 on whom data were published in 1982).

The parents of the index 29 children were asked to describe in some detail the developmental concerns that had first prompted them to consult a physician. Eight of the 29 families reported that they had consulted a physician regarding either their child's behavior or their child's development before the

Table 13
Presenting complaints

Complaint	Group 1		Group 2	
	N	%	N	%
Speech delay	15/21	71[a]	8/26	31
Withdrawal, preoccupation (including perseverative play)	10/21	48	8/26	31
Slow learner	6/21	29	6/26	23
Hyperactivity	4/21	19	6/26	23
Temper tantrums, negativism	3/21	14	5/26	19
Phobias	2/21	10	4/26	15
Thought disorder	2/21	10	3/26	12
Hallucinations, delusions	2/21	10	3/26	12
Incoherence	1/21	5	4/26	15

Note. The derivation of Group 1 and Group 2 is explained in Chapter 5.
[a] $p < .01$.

end of the second year of life. Three of the eight families approached their physician with motor concerns (poor muscle tone, no moving about, no grasping, poor chewing); four more brought concerns regarding the child's social responsivity ("he doesn't listen, he doesn't seem to care if I'm there or not")— two of these four also reported the infant to be extremely fearful; and the eighth child presented with severe nightmares during the first year of life and was investigated for a sleep disorder or a seizure disorder (the findings were negative; see description of this case in Chapter 2).

By the end of the fourth year of life, 11 more of the 29 children had presented to physicians with developmental or behavioral concerns. Lack of speech was by far the most common complaint, dominating the presentation of seven of these 11 cases. In three more cases the parents were concerned about "a loud voice and echoing speech" and stated that the child was "slow to talk and express himself." Other parental complaints included: "crying for no reason," "he lives in his own world," "he ignores everybody, including me," "he giggles and laughs for no apparent reason, but he won't talk," perseverative play, hyperactivity, and temper tantrums.

The remaining 10 children were seen during the fifth or the sixth year of life, usually as a result of teacher concern and recommendation. All of these children were noted to be relating either poorly or not at all with their peer group. Five of the children were regarded as "slow" or were described as seeming "not to understand." Two children were believed to be "too passive." Three of these children "hated" school and demonstrated school avoidance behavior (both somatic complaints and an overt refusal to attend school). One child was described as "immature and disruptive." One child lived so much in his fantasy world and spent so much time relating his perseverative ideas to his teacher that she became alarmed regarding his ability to differentiate reality from fantasy, especially in view of the fact that he was a "loner."

EARLY DIFFERENTIAL DIAGNOSIS

When a child is seen with developmental concerns prior to the development of communicative speech, differential diagnosis is difficult. Once a conscientious physician has examined the child and been satisfied that the child has no developmental disorder of known etiology, the possible diagnoses that still remain are attention deficit disorder, developmental language disorders, severe learning disabilities, autism, and childhood schizophrenia (major affective disorders do also present in early childhood, but current wisdom teaches that, with the exception of "failure to thrive," which is a manifestation of anaclitic depression, the affective disorders are not usually complicated by major developmental disorder).

Differentiating Childhood Schizophrenia from Other Causes of Autism

Several factors help select even the mute "preschizophrenic" child from among the children suffering from other causes of autism:

1. There is no history of birth defect or organic insult sufficient to explain the clinical symptoms.

2. Even at age 3 or younger schizophrenic children make good eye contact when seeking need fulfillment and use gestures to indicate their needs (only three of our 29 index cases used neither gestural nor verbal means to secure their immediate needs).
3. Most preschizophrenic infants like and anticipate being picked up.
4. Most preschizophrenic infants and toddlers are interested in their environment and demonstrate normal curiosity.
5. Most preschizophrenic infants and toddlers show some affection toward their caretakers and seek intimate human contact when they are hurt or frightened.

(I recognize that there may be a group of schizophrenic children who never acquire speech and who therefore cannot be differentiated from the group of autistic children.)

Differentiating Childhood Schizophrenia from Attention Deficit Disorder, Discrete Learning Disability, and Developmental Language Disorder

During the fourth and fifth years of life, differentiating the verbal, agitated schizophrenic child from other developmentally disordered children can be a difficult task. All of the developmental disorders can present with hyperactivity and a short attention span. All may have an abundance of "soft" neurological signs in the absence of any focal neurological disease, and all may present with a mildly to moderately compromised birth and neonatal history. Few families admit to a history of mental illness, at least during the initial consultation.

There are nevertheless several factors that do help to differentiate the schizophrenic child from other developmentally disordered children:

1. Sleep disturbance is a common symptom in childhood schizophrenia by the third year of life.
2. The attention span of the schizophrenic child is *variable* rather than short; for example, the schizophrenic child

may attend for long periods of time to a perseverative activity such as rolling cars back and forth, rocking, jumping up and down, or assembling puzzles.

3. The behavior of the schizophrenic child is *variable* rather than constantly hyperactive; for example, there may be days on which the schizophrenic child is actually lethargic rather than hyperactive.

4. The disturbance in thought process described in this book (Chapters 5 and 6) is not observed in the nonpsychotic, developmentally disordered child.

Differential diagnosis becomes easier as the child matures and his or her thinking becomes more complex. It is wise to avoid using psychoactive stimulants until there is a reasonable certainty that the diagnosis is not childhood schizophrenia. Stimulants can be psychotogenic in vulnerable children. Many a schizophrenic child has in fact been referred for psychiatric consultation after the administration of methylphenidate not only failed to bring symptom relief but actually exacerbated the symptoms.

CHAPTER FIVE

SIGNS AND SYMPTOMS OF CHILDHOOD SCHIZOPHRENIC DISEASE

In the future it may be possible for a physician who is looking after a preschizophrenic infant to document the child's sleep behavior, social behavior, and unusual behaviors or fears as they arise, and a record may be kept of the sequence in which speech develops. But this type of "prospective" observation of schizophrenic children has, in the past, rarely been documented (Fish, 1977, 1986). It is therefore not yet possible to say with any kind of certainty in what order the symptoms of schizophrenic disease appear.

From the "retrospective" data that are available to us, it would seem that a disturbance in the child's arousal state (e.g., sleep disturbance and/or lethargy alternating with periods of normal activity or overactivity) is one of the earliest signs of neuropsychiatric dysfunction. Other early signs include unexplained irritability, intense moodiness, an unwavering interest in certain objects coupled with a remarkable disinterest in almost anything else, autonomic instability (hyperthermia, pallor, and dilated or pinpoint pupils that are slow to respond to changes in light), and a "short attention span" (by parental report). Photographs of preschizophrenic children suggest that loss of muscle tone may also be an early sign of developmental disturbance (see Chapter 2, Figure 1).

PHYSICAL SIGNS

Physical Characteristic Scale

We have known for some time now that by the time schizophrenic children are first seen in psychiatric consultation they have a number of physical characteristics in common (Cantor *et al.*, 1981, 1982). At least some of these characteristics appear to be age dependent (Cantor *et al.*, 1982). A significant correlation between the score on the Physical Characteristic Scale and the score on the Symptom Scale has now been observed over a large number of cases (Figure 3), as has the tendency of the children to divide themselves into two groups,* a group in whom the symptom score is high relative to the physical characteristic score (Group 1) and a group in whom the two scores are more nearly equal (Group 2) (Tables 14 and 15).

Examining the very young schizophrenic child requires much patience and tact. These children are often so fearful of being touched by strangers that by the time they have reached their fourth year even their own family physician has begun to avoid doing a physical examination. The consulting psychiatrist would be wise to leave the physical examination to the last few minutes of the initial visit. The cooperation of some of the children can be enlisted by initially allowing the child to attempt to do the measuring (while the doctor unobtrusively takes charge of the tape measure), and of course by inviting the child to first measure the doctor! Full instructions on how to score an individual child, as well as a sample score sheet and the two scales, can be found in Appendix A. The results of doing a physical examination on 54 schizophrenic children are reported by group (Table 14) and by age (Figures 4 and 5).

Hypotonia

All of our 54 subjects, with the exception of one latency-aged girl, one adolescent girl, and one adolescent boy, were hypotonic at the time they were first seen (Figure 4). Even these three normotonic youngsters showed signs of neuromuscular dysfunction (they did poorly on the Bruininks–Oseretsky Test of Neuromuscular Proficiency; see Chapter 6) and they were therefore included within this group of hypotonic schizophrenics.

For the physician who is concerned about overdiagnosing hypotonia because of its "subjectivity," observing the presence of

---

*To be assigned to Group 1, the difference between the raw score on the Physical Characteristic Scale and the raw score on the Symptom Scale had to be ≥3, and the difference between the weighted score on the Physical Characteristic Scale and the weighted score on the Symptom Scale had to be ≥16.

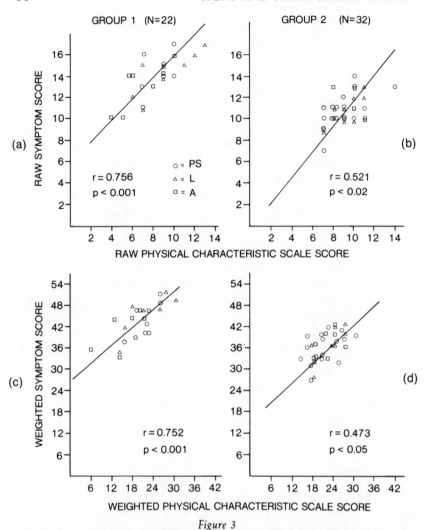

Figure 3

(a and b) The relationship between the raw score on the Physical Character-istic Scale and the raw score on the Symptom Scale for Group 1 and Group 2. (c and d) The relationship between the weighted score on the Physical Characteristic Scale and the weighted score on the Symptom Scale for Group 1 and Group 2.

Table 14
Incidence of physical signs

Characteristic	Group 1		Group 2	
	N	%	N	%
Physical Characteristic Scale				
Hypotonia	20/22	91	31/32	97
Brachycephaly	14/22	64	18/32	56
Long hands	9/22	41	12/32	38
Decreased muscle power	12/22	55	23/32	72
Decreased muscle mass	9/22	41	25/32	78[a]
Blue eyes	10/22	45	18/32	56
Hypercanthism ($>75\%$)	12/22	55	23/32	72
True hypercanthism ($>97\%$)	7/22	32	7/32	22
Soft velvety skin	18/22	82[b]	19/32	59
Head $>$ height	12/22	55	19/32	59
Increased head circumference ($>75\%$)	12/22	55	16/32	50
Prominent nasal bridge	7/22	32	12/32	38
Deep-set eyes	13/22	60	16/32	50
Short fingers	11/22	50	17/32	53
Lax elbows	8/22	36	17/32	53
Lax MCP joints and wrists	14/22	64	26/32	81
Mean number score	8.23 ± 2.27		9.13 ± 1.60	
Mean weighted score	20.23 ± 5.71		22.56 ± 4.09	
Associated physical characteristics				
Lordosis	14/22	64	23/32	72
Strabismus	4/22	18	8/32	25
Dysarthria	11/22	50	18/32	56
Flat feet	10/22	45	16/32	50
Loss of flexor tone	6/22	27	12/32	38
No arm swing while walking	14/22	64	14/32	44
Abnormal gait	18/22	82	25/32	78

[a]$p < .01$; [b]$p < .05$.

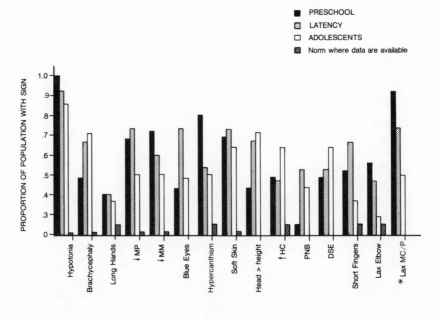

* Preschool more likely than adolescent (p <.005)

Figure 4
The results of using the Physical Characteristic Scale to assess three groups of childhood schizophrenics, preschoolers (aged 3–6), latency-aged children (aged 7–12), and adolescents (aged 13–18). Findings are reported by age group and are compared with normal values wherever such data are available.

"objective" signs (the associated signs listed in the bottom section of Table 14 and illustrated in Figure 5) of motor dysfunction should reinforce the clinical impression of poor resting tone.

Brachycephaly

The prevalence of brachycephaly tended to increase across age groups, being observed in less than half of the preschoolers and in almost 75% of the adolescents (Figure 4). Indeed, since I have been able to follow some of these youngsters for 7 years, I have had the opportunity to observe the development of brachycephaly in affected children who were between 4 and 8 years of age.

Long Hands

The prevalence of long hands within this population is slightly greater than within the nonschizophrenic population (36–40% of schizophrenic children have long hands compared with 25% of their age-matched peers; see Figure 4). As the study population increases in size, however, the prevalence of this finding appears to be regressing toward the normal mean (it had occurred in 80% of the pilot group; Cantor *et al.*, 1981).

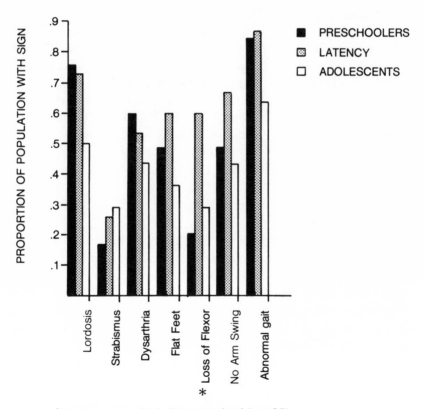

* Latency more likely than preschool (p < .05)

Figure 5
The results of documenting the associated physical signs on three age groups of childhood schizophrenics.

Decreased Muscle Power

Decreased muscle power was most frequently observed among latency-aged schizophrenic children (Figure 4). We have now had the opportunity to observe three children in whom muscle power weakened between the ages of 5 and 9 (despite ongoing gross motor therapy) and one child whose muscle power improved during puberty. This latter improvement may be temporary; this youngster once more became weaker as puberty receded and he entered the middle adolescent years.

Decreased Muscle Mass

Puberty is normally attended by an increase in muscle mass, even in 50% of schizophrenic individuals. We have recently begun enhancing the effect of normal maturation by enlisting schizophrenic adolescents in a weight-lifting program. In all the youngsters we have been able to persuade to try this program, muscle mass has increased most satisfactorily. In very young schizophrenic children the attenuation of muscle mass is best appreciated by looking for muscle contour. Lack of such contour has caused the arms of these children to be described as "tubular" (see Figure 6, a–d).

Blue Eyes

The increased prevalence of blue eyes in our pilot group prompted the speculation that this was yet another sign of dysmaturation in this population of children (the eyes of many blue-eyed babies darken with maturation). This finding may have been mere chance, however, because as the study group has enlarged, the prevalence rate has regressed toward the normal mean (Table 14).

Hypercanthism

Hypercanthism is very much more prevalent among preschool schizophrenic children than among the older childhood schizophrenic population (Figure 4), suggesting that it may correct itself with physical maturation. Nevertheless it remains significantly increased even among those childhood schizophrenics who have reached the adolescent years (occurring in 50% of adolescent childhood schizophrenics compared with 25% of their normal peers; see Figure 4). True hypercanthism (>97%) occurs in 10 times as many preschool schizophrenic children as in their age-matched peers (32% vs. 3%).

Soft Velvety Skin

The finding of soft velvety skin has remained fairly constant across age groups. It is most prevalent among those children and adolescents who have the highest symptom score (see Group 1 in Table 14). To the physician, the youngster's skin will feel like an infant's. The hyperesthesia (fear of touch or of labels on clothes) so frequently observed in this population may well be related to this unusual skin texture.

Head Greater than Height

A head circumference that was large relative to the child's height was more frequently observed among adolescent-aged childhood schizophrenics than in preschool or latency-aged subjects (Figure 4).

Increased Head Circumference

As with the other two "head" signs (brachycephaly and head greater than height), an increased head circumference was also most frequently observed in the adolescent-aged childhood schizophrenic population (Figure 4). An unusual head size and shape therefore appears to be the outcome of growth in a schizophrenic child, rather than an aberration occurring during the developing years.

Prominent Nasal Bridge

The finding of an unusually prominent nasal bridge is more common in the latency-aged and adolescent-aged schizophrenic child than in the preschooler (Figure 4). Except as part

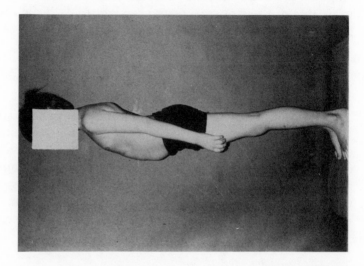

(a)

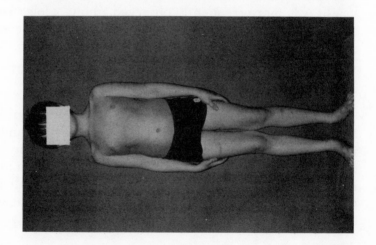

(b)

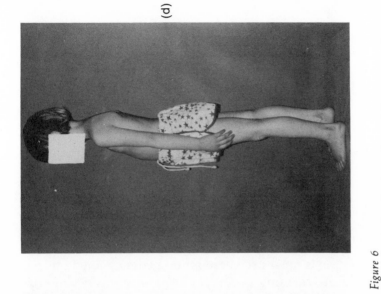

(d)

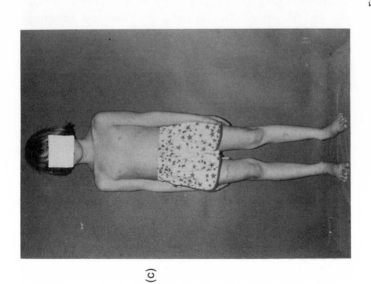

(c)

Figure 6

(a and b) Two views of a 9-year-old schizophrenic boy revealing lordosis, loss of flexor tone, decreased muscle mass (loss of muscle contour), and flat feet. (c and d) Two views of an 8-year-old schizophrenic boy revealing lordosis, loss of flexor tone, decreased muscle mass, and flat feet.

of a physiognomy cluster that appears to be associated with childhood schizophrenia, this finding probably has no clinical significance.

Deep-Set Eyes

The deep-set eyes of the schizophrenic child at any age are very striking. This finding also increases in prevalence with maturation (Figure 4). The children's eyes appear more sunken when they are ill. Many of these children resemble their allergic peers both in the appearance of their eyes and in the tendency to become very congested during infections of the upper respiratory tract (at least during the prepubertal years).

Short Fingers

This finding is most prevalent among latency-aged schizophrenic children, seeming to correct itself with physical maturation (Figure 4). A regression toward the normal mean is evident in the adolescent-aged childhood schizophrenics, in whom the finding occurs in 36% of the population, compared with 25% of their age-matched peers.

Lax Elbows

Lax elbows are most commonly observed in the preschool schizophrenic child (Figure 4). Among the adolescents this finding is only slightly increased above the norm, as we have reported that we found lax elbows in 20% of the normal subjects whom we examined (Cantor et al., 1981).

Lax Metacarpal–Phalangeal (MCP) Joints

This is a very common finding in preschool schizophrenic children. The affected child's joints may tighten up with maturation, although this laxness was still a positive finding in almost half of the adolescents (Figure 4).

Associated Physical Characteristics

Lordosis

Poor posture is a constant observation in schizophrenic children across age groups (Figures 5 and 6). During the prepubertal years, a majority of the children are moderately to severely lordotic. During adolescence some of these children are very much at risk for scoliosis (two of the males who are here counted among the preschool and latency subjects are now, in adolescence, being treated for scoliosis), and others collapse their chest and stomach muscles in such a way that they begin to develop kyphosis of the thoracic spine.

Strabismus

Strabismus is, of course, not age dependent, although a weak or wandering eye has been known to correct itself with maturation. Several of these children required corrective surgery. Most did not. Simple eye patching sufficed in at least one case.

Dysarthria

The majority of schizophrenic children do outgrow articulation difficulties. The rule of thumb that we try to follow is to enlist the aid of a speech pathology specialist if the child still has an articulation defect at 6 years of age. Forty-three percent of the adolescent-aged childhood schizophrenics still had a noticeable speech defect (Figure 5).

Loss of Flexor Tone

Loss of flexor tone is a sign that is said to be present if, when the affected individual stands upright, the force of gravity fully or partially extends the arm (Figure 6). There can be no doubt that an individual who has lost flexor tone is severely hypotonic. In most cases, the arm is not thus extended, although if the arm is seen to flop clumsily during active locomotion (e.g., running), this sign should be regarded as present.

No Arm Swing While Walking

The loss of arm swing while walking can be commonly observed in the adult schizophrenic population (with or without psychotropic medication). It is somewhat more common during the latency years in childhood schizophrenics, and it tends to be increased among the Group 1 subjects (Table 14).

Abnormal Gait

The gait of schizophrenic children is highly individualized, although visibly abnormal in most cases (Figure 5, Table 14). Some children lunge from place to place, others walk cautiously but with a broad base, still others toe walk, and some have a disjointed gait or other odd movement (Cantor *et al.*, 1981).

Fluctuating Signs and Symptoms

Pallor, flushed cheeks, and a glittery- or glassy-eyed look are intermittent signs of childhood schizophrenia. These signs come and go, even in the same child. Thus, a child with schizophrenia may at one time appear pale and listless; at another, flushed and agitated. The same child's pupil size may, at times, be dilated and slow to respond to changes in light, and at other times, it may be contracted to a pinpoint and slow to react to light change. There may also be long periods of time during which skin color and pupil size are unremarkable.

Of interest also is the unpleasant smell that may, at times, emanate from the hair, perspiration, and urine of childhood schizophrenics. The smell comes and goes, some parents insisting that it is at its worst when the child is most psychotic. The smell is characteristic, and I have noted it on occasion emanating from adults with poor prognosis schizophrenic disease. (I remember well a young man admitted to the psychiatric unit at McMaster University in whom four attempts to wash the smell from his hair failed. The smell disappeared several days after admission, as the young man's mental status slowly improved.)

In Summary

The physical examination of schizophrenic children revealed few differences between Group 1 and Group 2 childhood schizophrenics (Table 14). In general, the Group 2 subjects tended to show more evidence of neuromuscular dysfunction, as decreased muscle power, decreased muscle mass, hypercanthism, lax elbows, lax MCP joints, and loss of flexor tone were all observed more frequently in Group 2 subjects than in Group 1 subjects (Table 14). Of the physical signs, only brachycephaly, true hypercanthism, soft velvety skin, deep-set eyes, and lack of arm swing while walking occurred more often in Group 1 subjects than in Group 2.

SYMPTOMS

No healthy person thinks of crystal water when his house is being swept away by a flood; nor will he think of water as a medium of transportation when he is thirsty.

But in the normal mind only those part concepts dominate the picture that belong to a given frame of reference. (Bleuler, 1911/1950, pp. 16 and 17)

Symptom Scale

The symptoms common to childhood schizophrenia have previously been described (Cantor, 1982; Cantor et al., 1981, 1982). Appendix A includes a sample score sheet that can be used for assessing an individual child.

Schizophrenic preschoolers are best assessed in an unstructured play situation, the evaluator being especially sensitive to the child's "touch" needs (some children feel safe only when a grown-up is very near, even touching; others insist that a safe distance be maintained at all times). Schizophrenic adolescents are best assessed in an unstructured interview, special care being taken by the evaluator to try to set the youngster at ease. The results of examining the same 54 children and adolescents whose physical signs and symptoms have been described are reported by group (Table 15) and by age (Figure 7; see also Figure 13 in the later section on associated symptoms).

Table 15
Incidence of symptoms

Symptom	Group 1		Group 2	
	N	%	N	%
Symptom Scale				
Constricted affect*	22/22	100	30/32	94
Perseveration*	22/22	100	31/32	97
Inappropriate affect*	18/22	82	22/32	69
Anxiety	21/22	95[a]	24/32	75
Fragmented thought*	19/22	86	23/32	72
Hyperacusis	14/22	64	19/32	59
Monotonous inflection	19/22	86	20/32	63
Loose associations*	19/22	86	25/32	78
Neologisms	8/22	36[b]	2/32	6
Echolalia	11/22	50	10/32	31
Illogicality*	19/22	86	25/32	78
Mannerisms	15/22	68	17/32	53
Facial grimacing*	18/22	82[c]	12/32	38
Perplexity	17/22	77	23/32	72
Autistic thinking	17/22	77[c]	11/32	31
Clang associations	10/22	45	9/32	28
Incoherence*	16/22	73	18/32	56
Seven or more core symptoms (*)	17/22	77[c]	5/32	16
Mean number score	13.91 ± 2.07[c]		10.78 ± 1.58	
Mean weighted score	43.91 ± 5.18[c]		36.47 ± 4.18	
Average age when scored	10.50 ± 4.98		7.86 ± 4.05	
	7 preschool		18 preschool	
	7 latency		8 latency	
	8 adolescents		6 adolescents	
Associated symptoms				
Ambivalence	12/22	55	14/32	44
Hallucinations	9/22	41	10/32	31
Delusions	6/22	27	5/32	16
Paranoid ideation	7/22	32	12/32	38
Poverty of speech	15/22	68[d]	11/32	34
Poverty of content of speech	19/22	86[c]	17/32	53
Developmental data				
Speech delay	17/21	81[c]	10/26	38
Motor milestone delay	7/21	33[e]	2/26	8
Birth and postnatal complications	5/21	24	11/26	42

[a]$p < .048$; [b]$p < .01$; [c]$p < .005$; [d]$p < .025$; [e]$p < .05$.

Constricted Affect

Only two of our 54 subjects demonstrated a normal affective range at the initial psychiatric interview (Table 15). Both of these children were, however, preoccupied with morbid fears and fantasies, and therefore cannot truly be said to be affectively normal. Assessed in the way in which mental status examinations are traditionally conducted (i.e., as "present status" examinations), both of these children did, however, appear to have normal affective range. In both these cases, affect that was inappropriate to context was also noted (see subsequent discussion).

Affect is severely constricted in most schizophrenic children. One mother, determined to improve her son's ability to express himself affectively, enlisted him in the family's

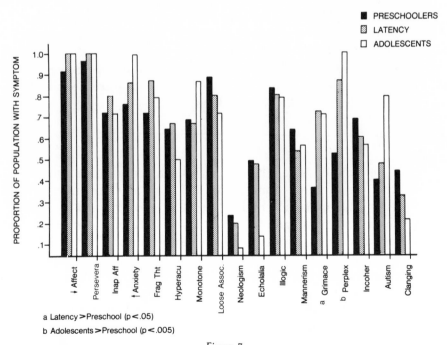

a Latency > Preschool (p < .05)

b Adolescents > Preschool (p < .005)

Figure 7

The results of using the Symptom Scale to assess three age groups of childhood schizophrenics.

professional clothes-modeling endeavors, defensively insisting that "the photographers taught him to smile" (the worried expression so characteristic of many schizophrenic children [see Chapter 2, Figure 2] was this little boy's dominant affect).

Perseveration

Only one of our 54 subjects betrayed no perseverative ideation during evaluation (Table 15). Even this child insisted on perseveratively examining every toy in my office and opening every enclosed object. She played with nothing.

Inappropriate Affect

The most common inappropriate affect observed in schizophrenic children is an incongruent smile or an inappropriate laugh. Projective play, when it occurs, is often violent, yet the child smiles throughout the play sequence even when the material being presented is clearly fearful (the accompanying words express the child's fear). Both parents and nursery school teachers have described affected children who appeared to be "laughing" at some "inner" joke yet were most unresponsive to external efforts to elicit a joyful response.

Anxiety

The fearfulness of the child with schizophrenia is not unlike the "pan-anxiety" long associated with adult forms of the disease. Schizophrenic children are easily frightened by that which is unfamiliar and which is associated with a moderate degree of sensory stimulation; for example, one child reacted to a talking toy telephone in my office with the words "I'm just a little girl!" as she hastily blocked off the telephone with a pile of wooden blocks.

Often the schizophrenic child's greatest fear seems to be not comprehending: One can observe the child's anxiety escalating in almost any situation that poses a cognitive challenge. Even 3-year-old schizophrenic children habitually greet new information with the words "I can't!" and "It's too hard!"

Anxiety is most prevalent in the adolescent-aged childhood schizophrenic population (Figure 7), probably reflecting the stresses that are an intrinsic part of this phase of human development.

Fragmented Thought

From the child's fragmented language productions (e.g., words and phrases more often than sentences) it is difficult to be certain whether it is the affected child's thought processing that is fragmenting already learned material, or whether the disorganized verbalizations are the result of piecemeal perceptions. It is probable that in most children both information gathering (perception and observation) and information processing (cognition) are disordered.

Frequently schizophrenic children seem to observe only a part of that which is presented to them (Norman, 1954). Thus, when four illustrations of fruits in different states of preparation (Figure 8) were hung upon the classroom wall, a schizophrenic 6-year-old asked the teacher "Why did you hang a diamond on the wall?" The child had responded to the shape that resulted from the juxtaposition of the four drawings rather than to the actual content of the illustrations.

The difficulty schizophrenic children experience with processing that which has been observed is best revealed by the inappropriate associations the children produce during projective play. Sometimes these associations appear to result from perseveration; for example, a schizophrenic child may begin to build a car out of Lego and may continue to reach for Lego pieces long after the car is complete—pieces may be added that represent a jet engine ("now it's an airplane," the child rationalizes), the walls of a house ("the car–house can fly," the child says), and so forth, the associations becoming more and more bizarre if the play is allowed to proceed unstructured by the interviewer. The child may continue to build until an unrecognizable structure emerges, although as the object becomes increasingly difficult to explain, the child often begins to complain of fatigue and to ask when the session will be over. If the interviewer attempts to limit the child's play, the child may

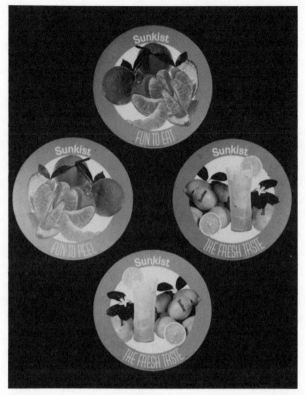

Figure 8

Four pictures of fruits in different stages of preparation were hung on the classroom wall by the director of our treatment program in order to encourage a more flexible approach to eating in the children (several of whom would reject food if it was presented in a new form). A schizophrenic child responded to the shape that the four pictures created on the wall ("Why did you hang a diamond on the wall?") rather than to the context of the pictures.

express perplexity, complain of fatigue, or become negative and insist that the bizarre structure is OK because "it's just pretend."

Hyperacusis

The inability to priorize incoming auditory information is termed "hyperacusis." The affected child or adolescent comments on sounds that are occurring down the hall or outdoors.

In extreme cases the child may be totally distracted by extraneous noise. This symptom is slightly less prevalent among adolescent-aged childhood schizophrenics (Figure 7), suggesting that maturation may improve the child's ability to selectively attend to sensory stimuli.

Monotonous Inflection

An unusually loud (or soft) voice that totally lacks affective expression is characteristic of the childhood schizophrenic. This difficulty in achieving vocal emotional expressivity may be even more evident in the childhood schizophrenic postpubertally, although even in very young children the mechanical quality of the child's voice frequently excites much comment.

Loose Associations

Latency- and adolescent-aged schizophrenic children frequently put their disordered thoughts down on paper (Figures 9 and 10). The child who is preliterate can provide many examples of a loosening in the associative process during an unstructured play session; for example, a 6-year-old who was drawing a picture of a graveyard and describing an accident he had witnessed suddenly remarked "My mom and I forgot to have our Halloween party." A 5-year-old remarked while playing with a toy house: "What's wrong in this house . . . it's just digged up like snow . . . that means it's dirty . . . somebody didn't clean it up" as he gazed at the house with a perplexed look.

Neologisms

Although many word approximations are heard during a play session with a schizophrenic child, neologisms are relatively rare (Figure 7 and Table 15). Schizophrenic children frequently introduce words that they have heard on television, and these may not be recognized by the examining psychiatrist. Before deciding a word is a neologism it is therefore important to be sure that the word has not been borrowed from the Saturday morning television cartoons.

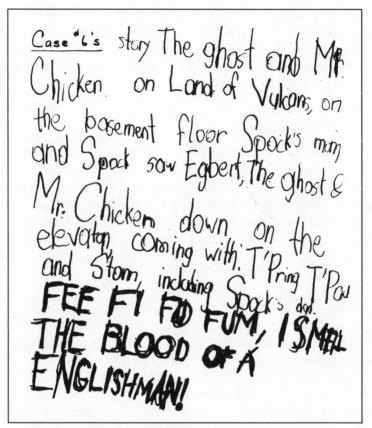

Figure 9

A spontaneous effort by a latency-aged schizophrenic child to write a story reveals condensation (as material from *Star Trek* and a children's story are condensed together), clang associations, and incoherence.

A few children write neologisms on their paperwork, easing the task of the examining psychiatrist (Figure 11). If one asks the child the meaning of the word, the reply will be a shrug or a perplexed look. The word appears to have no meaning even for the child who produced it.

Echolalia

During the initial phase of language development (a phase which may last 2–3 years in a schizophrenic child), many preschizophrenic children echo a part of every sentence directed their way. As language proficiency improves the children usually echo only that which they fail to comprehend. However, schizophrenic children may continue to echo as a way of showing their opposition to a command they do not wish to obey or their anger with a concept that they do not like or have misunderstood.

"Delayed echolalia" is a descriptive term for the child's tendency to reproduce exactly words heard either in everyday life or on television. It is not unusual for schizophrenic children to utter very adult phrases that are echos of the parent or guardian (the child uses the words out of context and obviously does not comprehend what he or she is saying). Occasionally delayed echolalia may be appropriate to the context of the situation; for example, a schizophrenic 8-year-old sang "you deserve a break today" (a phrase from a contemporary TV commercial) when he overheard two staff members discussing upcoming vacations!

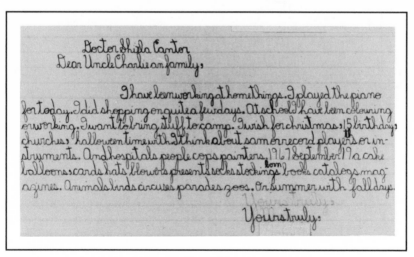

Figure 10
A 15-year-old childhood schizophrenic (documented history begins at age 6) attempts to write a letter to her therapist. The letter reveals loose associations and clang associations, and finally deteriorates into total incoherence.

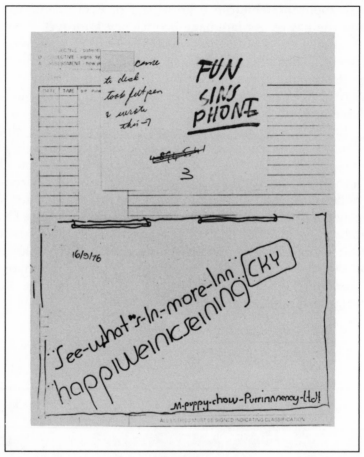

Figure 11
Spontaneous writing by a 9-year-old schizophrenic boy reveals a neologism.

Illogicality

The schizophrenic child is frequently illogical—and negative—that is, unlike a normal child who when corrected will shrug and accept the correct information, the schizophrenic child usually responds to corrections with an emphatic "No!" and perseverates with his or her own concept. An example is the 4-year-old schizophrenic child who enacted a play sequence in which the mother doll was first going shopping and then suddenly fell off a cliff; when told there were no cliffs in the middle of a shopping center, he angrily insisted it was so (it was evident the entire sequence was an intrusion from television cartoons because the child had never seen a cliff in reality).

The observations of schizophrenic children are frequently illogical; for example, a 6-year-old boy, after watching a ball bouncing off the wall, stated "We can't see the walls bouncing off." Another 6-year-old commented "Today I missed recess because some days we have recess and some days we don't" (he had in fact missed recess in order to keep his appointment with the therapist, and when that was pointed out to him he acknowledged that he was aware of that fact).

It is difficult for schizophrenic children to accept the multiple meanings of words; for example, a 9-year-old boy hit his play therapist after she stated that the sun was "hitting" the slate. He relaxed only after it was explained that "no, the sun does not have a fist." The same child had objected to the use of the term "stretcher" for the stretcher used to carry the sick and injured to an ambulance (he took a rubber band from my desk, called it a "stretcher," and demanded to know what it had in common with the ambulance equipment).

Mannerisms

The most common mannerisms observed in young schizophrenics are respiratory (e.g., clicking, blowing, etc.). In the latency- and adolescent-aged childhood schizophrenic, motor tics are more common. Hand mannerisms are infrequent, but they do occur in schizophrenics of all ages.

Facial Grimacing

The usual facial expression of a schizophrenic child is a puzzled frown. A scowling look is also frequently seen, however, as is an exaggerated squint or a grimacing smile. Grimacing is more prevalent among latency-aged and adolescent-aged childhood schizophrenics (Figure 7), occurring relatively rarely in the preschool childhood schizophrenic population.

Perplexity

As the ability of schizophrenic children to focus on the external world improves, their apparent puzzlement over what they see and hear becomes more evident (Figure 7). Their lack of comprehension extends to all spheres: social, cognitive, recreational, sexual, and so on. If they have been well treated and are trusting they will acknowledge their difficulties with constant demands to know: "why?" "what does that mean?" and "I don't understand."

Autistic Thinking

A preoccupation with self and with internal stimuli is observed with increasing frequency as the children mature (Figure 7). Even very young schizophrenic children occasionally think self-referentially: A 5-year-old girl, when told in answer to her inquiry as to the source of a noise that the wind was rattling the window, replied: "I didn't know there was wind outside." And a 5-year-old boy who had just witnessed a car accident involving a nearby car asked: "Mommy, did we hurt that car?"

"Clang" Associations

Untreated, schizophrenic children may continue to clang well into the latency years. Clanging may be evident when childhood schizophrenics free associate on paper (Figure 9) or in the classroom; for example, an 8-year-old wrote the words "group the grass" on the blackboard, then stood back and asked the therapist what it meant! A 5-year-old sang out "Hi, hi, back in the pie!" as he parked a toy car in the playhouse garage. Even in later years when adolescent childhood schizophrenics attempt to write paragraphs or compositions, clang associations may occur (Figure 10).

Incoherence

Incoherence is more common during the preschool years, as childhood schizophrenics appear to be better able to organize their language production as they mature (Figure 7). Most of the adolescent childhood schizophrenics are incoherent only when they are stressed or fatigued, or when they are confronted with a language assignment that is beyond their level of comprehension (Figure 12).

Associated Symptoms

Ambivalence

True ambivalence demands complex thinking; that is, one must be capable of simultaneously thinking two mutually conflicting thoughts or ideas. Hence, ambivalence is rarely observed in preschool schizophrenic children and is commonly observed in adolescent childhood schizophrenics (Figure 13). Occasionally ambivalence is revealed through the play of a young schizophrenic; for example, a 6-year-old playing with cars in my office remarked: "I wish it won't crash . . . it's s'posed to crash here."

Ambivalence can be very severe in childhood schizophrenics, extending to volition and to the motor apparatus: One 14-year-old routinely required half of our psychotherapy time to decide which game we should play; and a 16-year-old often lost motor control and began walking back and forth, getting on and off buses, and so on.

Hallucinations

Hallucinations are rarely described by preschool schizophrenic children, although we have frequently suspected that they were ongoing, and a few verbal preschoolers have been able to describe what they "saw" or "heard."* Thus one child anxiously insisted that Mickey Mouse was standing on the road in front of his father's car and that his father must not run him over! Another preschooler described "the walls

---

*An adult schizophrenic patient of mine recently described her "voices" to me thus: "Voices are different from my thoughts because I 'hear' the voices. I can even recognize whose voice it is, for example, my mother, a friend. . . . What makes it so weird is that the voices are inside my head, not outside!"

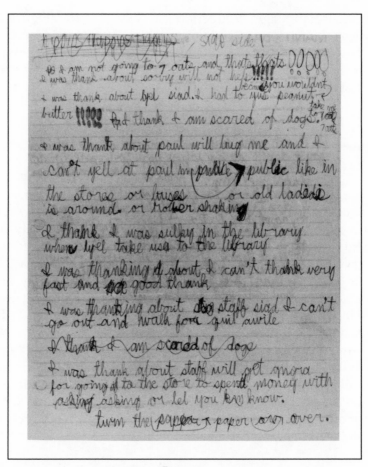

Figure 12

A 16-year-old schizophrenic boy (documented history begins at age 3) becomes totally disorganized in response to a demand that has been placed upon him by the staff of his group home. His spontaneous writing reveals fragmentation of thought processes, loose associations, high anxiety, and incoherence.

breathing" and the "funny lines that I see." Still another 5-year-old child cried and refused to be comforted, insisting that he could hear "noises and voices in my head."

During puberty hallucinations can become very troublesome to the childhood schizophrenic. One 15-year-old responded to a vocational teacher's comment on how music would improve the classroom by loudly proclaiming "I hear music in my head all the time . . . and voices too!" This youngster was so troubled by voices at 12 and 13 years of age that he asked his doctor for medication (this child's first 11 years are described in some detail elsewhere; Cantor, 1982).

Somatosensory hallucinations also occur in schizophrenic children. One 5-year-old frequently complained of "itchiness" (which caused him to squirm, not scratch) across his shoulders. These "sensations" were relieved when we put weights on his wrists (we hoped that by increasing the sensory input from his wrists, we would inhibit whatever it was he was perceiving across his shoulders).

Delusions

Like ambivalence, delusions require a complexity of thought process that is rarely observed in preschool schizophrenic children (Figure 13). We have therefore regarded this sign as present in preschoolers on only two occasions: a child who insisted he was the poison ivy exterminator (and who insisted that he could touch and play with poison ivy, resulting in frequent trips to a children's hospital emergency room), and a child who insisted he was more capable at any task than any grown-up (this child demonstrated his superiority by killing birds with his bare hands by the time he was 6 years old).

In latency, and even in early adolescence, the delusions that are seen in childhood schizophrenia continue to be primarily delusions of identity: for example, an 8-year-old who insisted he was an eggplant for a few weeks (after reading a story in which vegetables were anthropomorphized), a 14-year-old who was convinced he was the Incredible Hulk, another 14-year-old who was convinced she was married to a rock star, and so forth.

Paranoid Ideation

The conviction that one is being observed or controlled is far more common in the adolescent childhood schizophrenic. The preschooler lacks the cognitive sophistication to formulate such a concept (Figure 13). More frequently the young paranoid schizophrenic believes he can control others. It is not

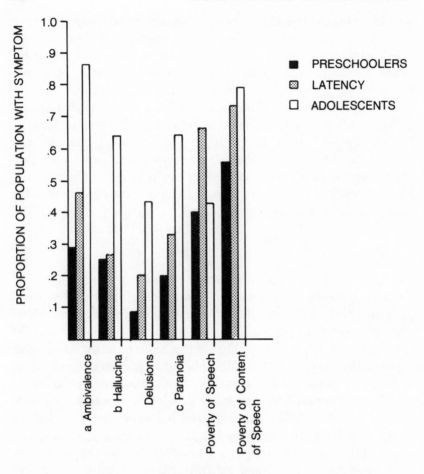

a Adolescents > Preschool (p < .004)
b Adolescents > Preschool (p < .05)
c Adolescents > Preschool (p < .04)

Figure 13

The results of documenting the associated symptoms on three age groups of childhood schizophrenics.

unusual to see a 5-year-old paranoid schizophrenic attempting to control every move of those about him. The 5-year-old "poison ivy exterminator" convinced an entire group of psychotic youngsters to join him in eliminating the offending poison ivy from the hospital grounds (there was, of course, no poison ivy growing there)!

Poverty of Speech

One-word answers and a lack of spontaneous communication are characteristic of many schizophrenic children. This symptom is most prevalent in the latency-aged childhood schizophrenic (Figure 13). The children become somewhat more verbal as a result of the "cognitive spurt" that attends adolescence.

Poverty of Content of Speech

The fragmented perceptions already described, the constant perseveration, and the anxiety with which new experiences are met ensure that poverty of content of speech will be manifest in childhood schizophrenics of all ages. As schizophrenic children are better treated and better educated, the severity of this symptom may be somewhat attenuated, although the prevalence is likely to remain high as a result of the defect in the associative process that is so central to this disease (Bleuler, 1911/1950).

In Summary

The core symptoms of childhood schizophrenia are significantly more prevalent within the Group 1 population, who also are more likely to manifest high anxiety, monotonous inflection, neologisms, echolalia, mannerisms, autistic thinking, and clang associations (Table 15). By almost every criterion used, the Group 1 children appeared to be "sicker" than the Group 2 children, despite the fact that a history of birth and postnatal complications was more common in Group 2 than in Group 1.

CHAPTER SIX

NEUROMUSCULAR AND COGNITIVE FUNCTIONING OF SCHIZOPHRENIC CHILDREN

Although the population of childhood schizophrenics does not appear to be functionally homogeneous, all of the affected children and adolescents have some signs of neuromuscular and cognitive dysfunction. In order to gain a more complete understanding of the specific strengths and deficits associated with this syndrome, we compared the performance of a group of affected children and adolescents on standardized tests of neuromuscular functioning with the level of achievement attained by the same (wherever possible) subjects on standardized psychometric tests.

TESTS OF NEUROMUSCULAR FUNCTIONING

The test that we used to assess motor functioning, the Bruininks–Oseretsky Test of Motor Proficiency (B-O), consists of tasks that are familiar or not difficult for a child to learn. It is therefore relatively easy to administer. Even those schizophrenic children who had spent most of their developing years in treatment facilities had had a great deal of exposure to many of the tasks included in the test, such as sit-ups or ball throwing.

The B-O consists of eight subtests: four of gross motor functioning, one of upper limb coordination, and three of fine motor functioning. Each subject tested is assigned a gross motor standard score, a fine motor standard score, and a battery composite standard score (a score based on the cumulative result of the gross motor, fine motor, and upper limb coordination subsections). An instruction manual is provided with the test materials; this describes in detail how to administer the test and includes full information on the standardization of scoring (Bruininks, 1978).

We tested the children and adolescents very slowly and over a period of several sessions. Care was taken to elicit the best possible performance from each subject so that a reliable measure of performance would be recorded. Four of the subjects (two from Group 1 and two from Group 2) were tested after almost 3 years of gross motor therapy.

We have tested 27 of the 54 childhood schizophrenics whose symptoms and signs are described in Chapter 5. Analysis of the data revealed no significant differences in performance between children and adolescents or between males and females (the number of females is too small for such differences to be revealed); therefore, the data are presented by subtest (Figure 14), in sum (Figure 15), and by group (Table 16).

Tests of Gross Motor Functioning

Running Speed and Agility

This test involves a short run (15 yards) on a straight track. Fifty-seven percent of the Group 1 subjects and 64% of the Group 2 subjects scored at least 1 standard deviation below the normal mean* on this subtest (Figure 14). Fifteen of the 27 subjects obtained their lowest test results on this subtest (eight from Group 1 and seven from Group 2). Despite the short running distance, many of the youngsters were breathless at the end of the test. Most maintained their arms in a fixed, abducted position while running. A few moved the trunk from side to side, contributing to the observed awkwardness of the run.

Balance

Eight items make up this subtest: (1) standing on preferred leg on floor; (2) standing on preferred leg on balance beam; (3) standing on preferred leg on balance beam—eyes

*The normal mean on the Bruininks–Oseretsky is 12. One standard deviation equals 5 points.

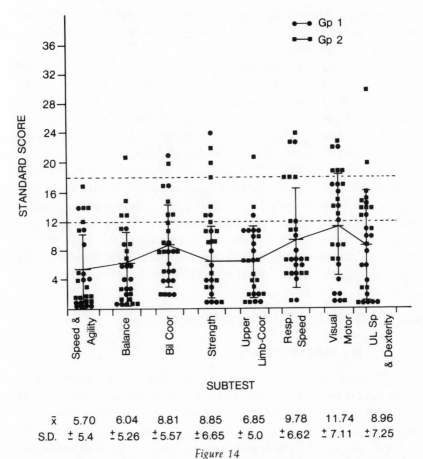

| x̄ | 5.70 | 6.04 | 8.81 | 8.85 | 6.85 | 9.78 | 11.74 | 8.96 |
| S.D. | ± 5.4 | ±5.26 | ±5.57 | ±6.65 | ± 5.0 | ±6.62 | ±7.11 | ±7.25 |

Figure 14

The results of testing using the Bruininks–Oseretsky are reported for Groups 1 and 2.

closed; (4) walking forward on walking line; (5) walking forward on balance beam; (6) walking forward heel-to-toe on walking line; (7) walking forward heel-to-toe on balance beam; and (8) stepping over response speed stick on balance beam. Eighty-four percent of the Group 1 subjects and 54% of the Group 2 subjects scored at least 1 standard deviation below the mean on this subtest (Figure 14). Nine of the 27 subjects obtained their lowest subtest score on this test (four from Group 1 and five from Group 2). Only one child, a 6-year-old, did really well on this subtest. Even this child was unable to perform item 3 successfully. No subject was able to stand on the balance beam more than 3 seconds with eyes closed, suggesting that balance might be impaired when the eyes could not be used. The last item, a test that requires a postural readjustment, was failed by most of our subjects.

Several of the children and adolescents tested internally rotated their legs and adducted their knees in a tightly locked position in an attempt to compensate for poor trunk control. Adventitious movements, such as grimacing or tightening of fists accompanied by arm flexion, were often observed during the balance subtests, as were poorly coordinated, thrashing-like movements of the arms. Some children appeared unable to close their eyes independently of other facial motor movements (resulting in a grimace). Some children reacted fearfully or negatively

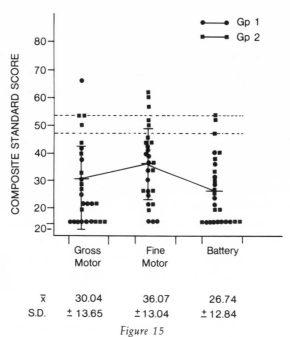

	Gross Motor	Fine Motor	Battery
x̄	30.04	36.07	26.74
S.D.	± 13.65	± 13.04	± 12.84

Figure 15

The composite standard scores achieved on the Bruininks–Oseretsky by Groups 1 and 2.

Table 16
Some parameters of neuromuscular function

Subtest	Group 1 ($N = 13$)	Group 2 ($N = 10$)
Running speed and agility	4.31 ± 4.37	6.21 ± 12.62
Balance[a]	4.38 ± 3.12	7.57 ± 6.41
Bilateral coordination	7.31 ± 5.60	10.21 ± 5.28
Strength	6.69 ± 6.54	10.86 ± 6.33
Upper level coordination	7.46 ± 4.41	6.29 ± 5.59
Response speed	7.0 ± 5.37	11.64 ± 7.33
Visual–motor	9.46 ± 7.29	13.86 ± 6.49
Upper limb speed and dexterity	5.69 ± 4.37	12.71 ± 7.45[b]
Gross motor composite standard score	27.0 ± 13.93	32.86 ± 13.24
Fine motor composite standard score	30.23 ± 8.94	41.5 ± 14.16[c]
Battery composite score	24.31 ± 8.68	31.86 ± 12.84

[a]Variance is significantly greater in Group 2 than in Group 1.
[b]$p < .008$.
[c]$p < .024$.

when asked to close their eyes while standing on the balance beam. Several of our subjects identified the balance beam as a task they feared, avoided, or always had trouble with at school.

Bilateral Coordination

Eight items make up this subtest: (1) tapping feet alternately while making circles with fingers; (2) tapping—foot and finger on same side synchronized; (3) tapping—foot and finger on opposite sides synchronized; (4) jumping in place—leg and arm on same side synchronized; (5) jumping in place—leg and arm on opposite sides synchronized; (6) jumping up and clapping hands; (7) jumping up and touching heels with hands; and (8) drawing lines and crosses simultaneously. The items are complex and are not mastered by a majority of normal children before the age of 9 years. Young schizophrenic children may therefore fail most of the items on this subtest and still compare favorably with the normal child (who also has not yet mastered these tasks). Of the 16 subjects in our cohort who were 9 years of age or older at the time of testing, only two received an average or above average score on this subtest. The other six subjects who achieved an "average" score (Figure 14) were all younger than 9 years.

Only the second item on this subtest was easily passed by a majority of our childhood schizophrenic subjects. Four of the remaining six pass–fail tests were failed by a majority of the prepubertal subjects and passed by a majority of the postpubertal subjects, suggesting that maturation may occur in some subjects in this aspect of functioning. Several of the adolescents directed themselves aloud as they performed many of the tasks of the bilateral coordination subtest.

Strength

Four items make up this subtest: (1) standing broad jump; (2) sit-ups; (3) knee push-ups (for boys under 8 and all girls); and (4) full push-ups (for boys age 8 and older). Seventy-six percent of the Group 1 subjects and 28% of the Group 2 subjects scored at least 1 standard deviation below the mean on this subtest (Figure 14). Three of the four preschoolers who had received intensive gross motor therapy achieved above average scores on this subtest, confirming our clinical impression that although therapy does not seem to improve resting motor tone, it does improve muscle strength and motor functioning.

The most difficult item for our subjects was usually the sit-ups. Subjects attempted to pull themselves up by grabbing their own pantlegs or by using their elbows. Several of the children and adolescents appeared to be unable to use their abdominal muscles. A few of the children were observed to have poor head control in the supine position. In the push-ups, some of the adolescents slammed their bodies into the mat, appearing to be unable to regulate this movement.

Tests of Upper Limb Coordination

This section of the B-O consists of a single subtest composed of 9 items: (1) bouncing a ball and catching it with both hands; (2) bouncing a ball and catching it with preferred hand;

(3) catching a tossed ball with both hands; (4) catching a tossed ball with preferred hand; (5) throwing a ball at a target with preferred hand; (6) touching a swinging ball with preferred hand; (7) touching nose with index fingers—eyes closed; (8) touching thumb to fingertips—eyes closed; and (9) pivoting thumb and index finger. The performance of our subjects was the most homogeneous on this subtest and, in at least six cases, the most impaired. Forty-six percent of the Group 1 subjects and 79% of the Group 2 subjects scored at least 1 standard deviation below the mean on this subtest (Figure 14). Although the items on this subtest should be performed with ease by older children (they are really not demanding enough), only one adolescent performed in an above average manner. Item 7 was the only item on this subtest that was easily passed by a majority of the older subjects, although very young schizophrenic children had considerable difficulty with this item.

The difficulty schizophrenic children experience with upper limb coordination may have major social consequences, because the ability to engage in ball play is central at many social interactions in middle childhood. When schizophrenic children first enter treatment they frequently respond to a tossed ball with a defensive reaction (a "startle"). Without gross motor therapy such children either totally avoid ball play or continue to use both hands to both catch and throw a ball until 9 or 10 years of age.

Tests of Fine Motor Functioning

Response Speed

This test involves a simple measure of how rapidly the subject interrupts the fall of a yardstick. The test was relatively well performed by most of our subjects, perhaps because the actual motor components of this subtest is minimal (it requires only the ability to tap one's thumb). Most of the younger subjects appeared to enjoy this task, once it had become familiar (Figure 14). Only two subjects, both adolescents, were too slow to respond (for one of these subjects, a boy who actually scored above our median on the battery composite standard score, his performance on this task was one of his two lowest subtest scores).

Visual–Motor Control

This subtest is composed of eight items: (1) cutting out a circle with preferred hand; (2) drawing a line through a crooked path with preferred hand; (3) drawing a line through a straight path with preferred hand; (4) drawing a line through a curved path with preferred hand; (5) copying a circle with preferred hand; (6) copying a triangle with preferred hand; (7) copying a horizontal diamond with preferred hand; and (8) copying overlapping pencils with preferred hand. Nine of our 27 subjects achieved their highest score on this subtest, as 54% of the Group 1 subjects and 79% of the Group 2 subjects demonstrated average or better performance on this subtest (Figure 14). Very young schizophrenic children, even those who had received intensive therapy, experienced much difficulty with Items 1 and 4.

This test provides an excellent opportunity to observe the ambidexterity of schizophrenic children (which in untreated children may persist until 8 or 9 years of age) as well as the difficulty many of these children experience with crossing the midline and with motor planning; for example, most schizophrenic children need to be told to steady the paper with the nondominant hand, and many will switch hands whenever a task demands crossing the midline. The occasional schizophrenic child, at last one in this group of 27 youngsters, is a truly gifted artist. It was interesting to observe that even this child, who drew so exceptionally well, utilized an immature pencil grasp.

Upper Limb Speed and Dexterity

This subtest is composed of eight items: (1) placing pennies in a box with preferred hand; (2) placing pennies in two boxes with both hands; (3) sorting shape cards with preferred hand; (4) stringing beads with preferred hand; (5) displacing pegs with preferred hand; (6) drawing vertical lines with preferred hand; (7) making dots in circles with preferred hand;

and (8) making dots with preferred hand. Sixty-nine percent of Group 1 subjects, but only 21% of Group 2 subjects, scored at least 1 standard deviation below the mean on this subtest (Figure 14). Three of the 11 subjects who had achieved average or better scores on this subtest were within the group of four children who were tested after 3 years of gross motor therapy. Even these children experienced considerable difficulty with Items 3 and 4 of this subtest.

Several of the prepubertal subjects seemed uncertain how to hold the deck of cards. During the stringing of beads (especially by children in whom other signs of mixed dominance were observed), the "assist hand" tended to be confused with the hand that was required to do the more precise movements, or a child would waste time moving each bead to the end of the string before placing the next bead, thus reducing his or her test score. Even children and adolescents who had had ample time to practice continued to perform these tasks more slowly than their peers.

Intertest Variability

The performance of our childhood schizophrenic subjects on the B-O tended to be highly variable: 17 of our 27 (63%) subjects demonstrated a subtest score range of 12 or more points; that is, for 17 of our children and adolescents the difference between the lowest and the highest subtest score was 12 or more points (2 standard deviations).

Comparison between Gross Motor and Fine Motor Functioning

As a group, both Group 1 and Group 2 childhood schizophrenics had less difficulty with the fine motor portion of the B-O than with the gross motor portion (Table 16 and Figure 15). Thus, nine of our 27 subjects were "unscorable" (achieved a composite score of −20) on the gross motor section of the test, while only three of the 27 subjects were "unscorable" on the fine motor section. Seventeen of the 27 subjects received higher scores on the fine motor section of test than on the gross motor section. In 10 of these subjects the difference between the fine motor composite score and the gross motor composite score was 10 or more points (2 standard deviations).

Only eight of our subjects did better on the gross motor section than on the fine motor, and in only two cases was this difference significant (10 or more points). Three of these eight subjects (including the two in whom the difference between the gross motor composite score and the fine motor composite score achieved statistical significance), were the children who had received intensive gross motor therapy.

In Summary

Few differences emerged between the Group 1 and Group 2 subjects on these standardized tests of neuromuscular functioning. As a group the Group 2 children did better than the Group 1 children on all subtests except upper limb coordination (Figures 14 and 15 and Table 16). The difference in performance between the two groups reached statistical significance only on tests of fine motor functioning (Table 16). At least in this area of functioning, the Group 2 children demonstrated once again that they are less impaired than the Group 1 children.

TESTS OF COGNITIVE FUNCTIONING

Of the 54 childhood schizophrenics who are described in Chapter 5, 24 have been assessed, using the Wechsler Intelligence Scale for Children—Revised (WISC-R; Wechsler, 1974) in 23 cases and the Wechsler Adult Intelligence Scale (WAIS; Wechsler, 1955) in one case. Most of these childhood schizophrenics were testable, although the test results on the occasional youngster who had virtually no periods of lucidity were not considered to be valid (in some cases we delayed testing a child until after 2–3 years of treatment).

Special care was taken to ensure that each subject performed maximally. The testing was often spread over several sessions, and testing sessions were postponed if there was any exacerbation of psychosis. Since our preliminary data analysis revealed no differences that could be attributed to the age or the sex of the testee, each subject's best test results are reported by subtest (Figure 16), in sum (Figure 17), and as part of a group result (Table 17).

Verbal Subtests

Information

Forty-two percent of Group 1 subjects and 33% of Group 2 subjects scored at least 1 standard deviation below the normal mean* on the Information subtest (Figure 16). In part, this result reflected the education of our subjects, as one adolescent had been at home since age 7 with no education input, three children had only special education, five children had been floundering in the mainstream with no resource help, and the remaining children and adolescents had had a combination of mainstreaming, resource help, and special education (after all else had failed).

Similarities

Forty-nine percent of the Group 1 subjects and 49% of the Group 2 subjects scored at least 1 standard deviation below the normal mean on the Similarities subtest (Figure 16).

Thought disorder interfered with the subjects' performance on this subtest as some children clanged in response to questions on similarity, others perseverated on a theme that had been initiated during a previous question, and still others derailed and responded with answers that revealed the occurrence of condensation.

Thus, when asked "What is alike about a wheel and a ball?" a 13-year-old clanged "wall" (a response that could also be interpreted as a condensation of the words "ball" and "wheel," or as a derailment in which he associated "wall" with ball play).

*The normal mean on both the WISC-R and the WAIS is 10. One standard deviation equals 3 points.

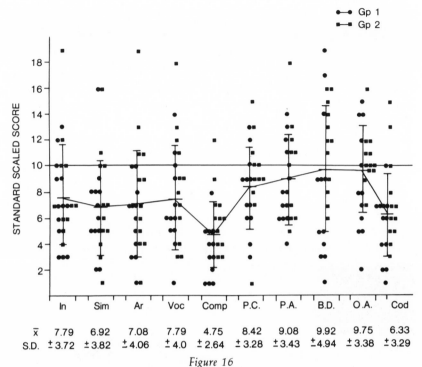

	In	Sim	Ar	Voc	Comp	P.C.	P.A.	B.D.	O.A.	Cod
x̄	7.79	6.92	7.08	7.79	4.75	8.42	9.08	9.92	9.75	6.33
S.D.	±3.72	±3.82	±4.06	±4.0	±2.64	±3.28	±3.43	±4.94	±3.38	±3.29

Figure 16

The results of testing using the WISC-R are reported for Groups 1 and 2.

In response to the question "In what way are a candle and a lamp alike?" an 8-year-old boy replied "A candle is a dynamite." Further questioning prompted the child to volunteer that a candle and a dynamite had the same thickness. The child made no attempt to answer the stated question regarding the similarity between the candle and the lamp. The same child responded to the question "In what way are a wheel and a ball alike?" with "Kick the ball, dynamite" as he perseverated on the dynamite theme.

Negativism and perplexity were also frequently revealed during this subtest. One 16-year-old girl, when asked to reply to three questions regarding similarity, "mountain–lake, first–last, and 49–121," looked puzzled and replied flatly "They are not alike."

Arithmetic

Fifty-eight percent of Group 1 subjects and 41% of Group 2 subjects scored at least 1 standard deviation below the normal mean on this subtest (Figure 16). As with the Information subtests, the effect of education upon each subject's performance in this subtest must be considered. Schizophrenic youngsters tend to perseverate upon concepts that have been mastered and to resist the introduction of new concepts. Few teachers persist with the introduction of new concepts.

Vocabulary

Fifty-eight percent of Group 1 subjects and 32% of Group 2 subjects scored at least 1 standard deviation below the normal mean on this subtest (Figure 16).

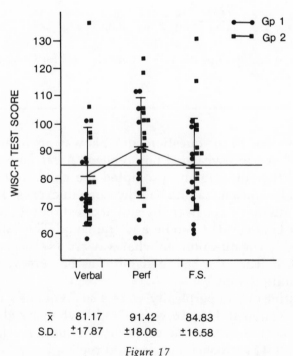

	Verbal	Perf	F.S.
$\bar{x}$	81.17	91.42	84.83
S.D.	±17.87	±18.06	±16.58

Figure 17
A summary of the scores on the WISC-R achieved by Groups 1 and 2.

Table 17
Results of testing on the WISC-R

Subtest	Group 1 ($N = 12$)	Group 2 ($N = 12$)
Information	6.75 ± 2.93	8.83 ± 4.24
Similarities	6.75 ± 3.70	7.08 ± 4.10
Arithmetic	5.92 ± 2.81	8.25 ± 4.86
Vocabulary	7.0 ± 3.49	8.58 ± 4.46
Comprehension	3.5 ± 2.11	6.0 ± 2.59[a]
Picture Completion	7.92 ± 3.0	8.92 ± 3.6
Picture Arrangement	8.5 ± 3.21	9.67 ± 3.68
Block Design	8.25 ± 5.75	11.58 ± 3.45
Object Assembly[b]	8.83 ± 4.17	10.67 ± 2.15
Coding	5.25 ± 2.67	7.42 ± 3.60
IQ		
Verbal	76.08 ± 11.82	86.25 ± 21.72
Performance	85.25 ± 19.33	97.58 ± 15.01
Full Scale	78.83 ± 13.21	90.83 ± 17.94

[a]$p < .018$.
[b]Variance is significantly greater in Group 1 than in Group 2.

The Vocabulary subtest often elicited clang associations from schizophrenic children and adolescents. Thus, when asked to define the word "belfry," a 15-year-old boy replied "bats in the belfry."

Tangential associations were also offered as definitions, and these could not be scored. Thus the word "contagious" was defined as "dangerous" by an 8-year-old, who also defined "migrate" as "join" and "alphabet" as a "bunch of words."

Poverty of speech was most in evidence during the Vocabulary and the Comprehension subtests. Thus, in reply to the question "What is espionage?" a 15-year-old boy replied simply "It's a crime."

Autistic logic (self-referential thinking) also revealed itself on this subtest, as a 15-year-old defined "brave" as "I am the greatest, I am a strong boy!" and "contagious" as "I am so contagious that I could blow my top off."

Comprehension

The WISC-R functioning of our subjects was the most homogeneous and the most depressed on this subtest, as

92% of Group 1 subjects and 66% of Group 2 subjects scored at least 1 standard deviation below the normal mean (Figure 16). Only one subject, a Group 2 adolescent, received an average score on this subtest. No subject, not even a child who had a Verbal IQ of 130 (despite a Verbal Comprehension subtest score of 7), demonstated above average functioning on this subtest. For 10 of the 14 subjects, Verbal Comprehension was the lowest subtest score achieved on the WISC-R.

Perplexity, poverty of speech, and total derailment were frequently observed during this subtest. Thus, when asked "What is the one thing for you to do when you cut your finger?" a 9-year-old replied, "With tweezers, with nail cutters, on elevator. Cry in an emotional response to cut or elevator."

When asked "What are you supposed to do when you find someone's wallet or pocket book in a store?" an 8-year-old replied "Make bullrushes out of it!"

Ambivalence also interfered with the ability of these subjects to successfully answer the questions on this subtest. In response to "Why is it usually better to give money to a well-known charity than to a street beggar?" a 16-year-old girl replied, "Charity can use it—a beggar can use it too."

Performance Subtests

Picture Completion

Thirty-three percent of Group 1 children and 25% of Group 2 children scored at least 1 standard deviation below the normal mean on this subtest (Figure 16). The greatest difficulties many subjects experienced with this, and with the other performance subtests, were difficulty attending to the task and a tendency to give up without trying simply because the material was new and unfamiliar.

Picture Arrangement

On this subtest as well, 33% of Group 1 subjects and 25% of Group 2 subjects scored at least 1 standard deviation below the normal mean (Figure 16).

Block Design

Fifty-one percent of Group 1 subjects scored at least 1 standard deviation below the normal mean on this subtest, but only 8% of Group 2 subjects did poorly on this subtest (Figure 16). In fact, 24% of Group 1 subjects and 33% of Group 2 subjects scored at least 1 standard deviation above the normal mean on this subtest. In eight of these 24 subjects, Block Design was the highest score achieved on the WISC-R.

Object Assembly

Thirty-three percent of the Group 1 subjects scored at least 1 standard deviation below the normal mean on this subtest, but none of the Group 2 subjects scored below the normal mean on this subtest (Figure 16).

Coding

The coding subtest presented considerable difficulty to both the Group 1 and the Group 2 subjects, as 58% of the Group 1 and 50% of the Group 2 subjects scored at least 1 standard deviation below the normal mean on this subtest (Figure 16).

The depressed functioning observed on the Coding subtest appeared to be a function of the time constraints placed upon the task; that is, most of the subjects were able to reproduce each symbol perfectly but produced too few symbols within the time limits of the task. A few subjects demonstrated perseveration of task, as they reproduced the same symbol over and over again instead of responding to the code.

Intertest Variability

Extreme variability in intellectual functioning has previously been described as characteristic of childhood schizophrenics (Wechsler & Jaros, 1965). This variability is revealed by the large number of children and adolescents in our cohort in whom the difference between the individual subject's own lowest subtest score and that same individual's highest subtest score is greater than 2 standard deviations. Ninety-two percent of Group 1 subjects and 83% of Group 2 subjects had such a subtest range. Indeed in 14 of 24 cases (six from Group 1 and eight from Group 2) that subtest range was greater than or equal to 3 standard deviations.

Most of our subjects achieved significantly higher scores on the Performance section of the WISC-R than on the Verbal section, as 25% of Group 1 subjects and 50% of Group 2 subjects had Performance minus Verbal scores of 16 or more points (Table 17 and Figure 17). Only one subject, a 6.5-year-old Group 2 child, did significantly better on the Verbal section of the WISC-R than on the Performance section (this was the child with the Verbal IQ of 130 mentioned earlier).

COMPARISON BETWEEN NEUROMUSCULAR AND COGNITIVE FUNCTIONING

A positive correlation was observed between the Full Scale WISC-R score and the B-O battery composite score (Figure 18), although considerable scatter exists (particularly with Group 2) and there were several "outliers" within the population of Group 2 subjects. Bruininks (1978) reported a similar correlation in normal children between the performance on the B-O and the WISC-R: The poorer the performance on the WISC-R, the poorer the performance on the B-O; in "normal" children, the corollary—that is, the better the performance on the WISC-R, the better the performance on the B-O—did not follow.

It is doubtful that performance on the B-O is a function of comprehension, since at least one child whose psychosis precluded psychometric testing was able to complete the motor testing, and a child with a Full Scale IQ of 130 showed major deficits in functioning on motor testing (this child scored more than 2 standard deviations below the mean on the balance and the upper limb coordination subtests of the B-O.)

The Group 2 subjects, who performed better than the Group 1 subjects in most areas of neuromuscular functioning (Table 16), approached normative functioning only on the response speed, visual–motor, and the upper limb speed and dexterity subtests; and on the fine motor composite standard

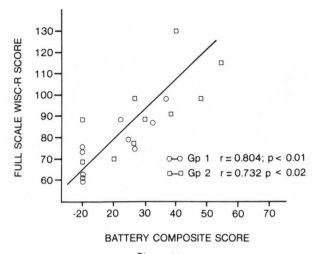

Figure 18

The correlation between neuromuscular functioning as measured by the Bruininks–Oseretsky and cognitive functioning as measured by the WISC-R is presented for Groups 1 and 2.

score. In all other areas of motor functioning, they scored significantly below the normal mean. The Group 1 subjects scored significantly below the normal mean in all areas of neuromuscular functioning tested.

Similarly in tests of cognitive functioning, the Group 2 subjects demonstrated average functional capacity on the Picture Arrangement, Block Design, and Object Assembly subtests; and on the performance subsection of the WISC-R (Table 17). All other areas of functioning revealed a mild to moderate depression in functioning. The Group 1 subjects revealed a mild to moderate depression in functioning in all areas of cognitive functioning tested.

A PROPOSED ORDER OF LOSS IN FUNCTIONAL CAPACITY

Despite the fact that a more global depression in functioning is observed in Group 1 subjects than in Group 2 subjects, the same pattern of "highs" and "lows" occurred in both populations (Tables 16 and 17). A pattern of loss of functioning, possibly related to the severity of the disease process in an individual subject, suggests itself: Gross motor functioning appears to be the first function to be depressed, followed by verbal intellectual functioning, followed by fine motor functioning, followed by the Performance aspects of the WISC-R. According to this working hypothesis: If Performance IQ is depressed, *all* areas of functioning should be depressed; if gross motor functioning is intact, *all* areas of functioning should be intact; and a depression of the Verbal IQ should precede the loss of fine motor functioning.

Thus, the two subjects (both from Group 2) who had demonstrated average or better gross motor functioning achieved average or better scores on fine motor functioning, and on both the Verbal and the performance sections of the WISC-R. Conversely, of the eight subjects (six from Group 1 and two from Group 2) who had achieved below average Performance IQ scores, all demonstrated a global loss in functioning. The only exceptions to this pattern of loss were two youngsters with both gross and fine motor deficits in functioning who had nevertheless maintained both Verbal and Performance IQs in the normal range.

The observed differences between Group 1 and Group 2 subjects also conform to this hypothetical pattern of function loss. Thus, the Group 2 subjects outperformed the Group 1 subjects on all measures of functioning except the Physical Characteristic Scale. In other words, even those subjects who were the least "sick" (the Group 2 subjects) did nevertheless have those signs of neuromuscular dysfunctioning that, according to the preceding suggestion, may be the earliest developmental loss to occur in childhood schizophrenia.

Thus, although signs of motor dysfunctioning in an adult with schizophrenia may be used as a sign of the childhood-type disease (see the Introduction), within the group of childhood schizophrenics, poor motor functioning does not indicate the severest end of the spectrum. Severity of disease, within the childhood schizophrenia population, is indicated by the presence of such symptoms as high anxiety, neologisms, facial grimacing, and autistic thinking (Table 15).

CHAPTER SEVEN

THE CASE FOR EARLY IDENTIFICATION AND TREATMENT

Schizophrenia is not a puberty psychosis in the strict sense of the word, although in the majority of patients the sickness becomes manifest soon after puberty. With relatively accurate case histories, one can trace back the illness to childhood, or even to the first years of life, in at least five per cent of cases. In this process we completely disregard the anomalies which do not have a distinctly schizophrenic character, although we know that the disease includes many symptoms of general significance.

At the present time we know of no differences between the infantile and other forms of the disease. If we observe patients during childhood, they present the same symptoms as those seen in adults. We did note, however, that the analyses of such youthful patients is more difficult. In contrast to adults, children are not less clear in their desires and wishes, but the content is less distinctly defined. The difficulty may also be due to our inadequate experience with the technique of handling youthful psychotics.—Bleuler (1911/1950, pp. 140 and 141)

The reluctance to identify "beautiful," "normal-looking" children as suffering from a chronic and disabling disorder has been described (see the Introduction). Many have argued that in the absence of a cure, "labeling" is unethical. The consequences of such reluctance to label have been eloquently described elsewhere by two parents whose children were not accurately identified (Spungen, 1983; Wilson, 1968). The apparent natural history of untreated childhood schizophrenia also suggests that a rethinking of the antilabeling position is in order.

CLINICAL COURSE OF UNTREATED
CHILDHOOD SCHIZOPHRENIA

Prospective studies of untreated versus treated childhood schizophrenics are not available. There are, however, retrospective anecdotal accounts that are illuminating.

It would seem that the moderately affected unidentified childhood schizophrenics "drop into" the mental retardation educational stream late in latency (Richards, 1951). (Here in Winnipeg we are now losing the severely affected unidentified childhood schizophrenics to mental retardation during the preschool years.) As deinstitutionalization has proceeded in Manitoba, I have been called to consult on a number of adult childhood schizophrenics, now aged 30 or older, some of whom had been placed in provincial institutions at 10 or 11 years of age. The biographical stories were remarkably similar: A child who had been late to talk, who had initially been regarded as an "anxious" slow learner, and who had been maintained in special education placements until behavior either in school or at home had become intolerable. Some families had gone from doctor to doctor seeking answers. A few had been told it was "developmental" and "might pass."

An acute exacerbation of psychotic symptoms—usually following a life-situation change such as deinstitutionalization, the death of a parent, aging parents who felt it was time for placement outside the home, and so on—has been the most frequent reason for consulting a psychiatry service in planning for childhood schizophrenics who had long since been integrated with the mentally handicapped. Typical presenting complaints have been severe agitation accompanied by irritable, threatening responses (a 16-year-old who pursued and proclaimed his "love" for a shopgirl; a 30-year-old who was in the process of moving from his parental home to a group home), "hallucinations" (an 18-year-old constantly addressing "the air" with laughter and with fear), and florid delusional thinking (a 16-year-old who believed she was pregnant; a 29-year-old who was convinced there was a world project dedicated to destroying her). A severe sleep disturbance usually accompanied the psychotic decompensation, and involved family members were able to confirm that they had encountered

both the behavior and the sleep disturbance during the identified patient's growing-up years. In all of these cases hospital
records of prepubertal consultation were available and a diagnosis of "autism" or "childhood schizophrenia" had been documented.

Among the adolescent-aged childhood schizophrenics
who are described throughout this book there are several
youngsters who presented and were identified as psychotic
during the preschool years, and who were "mainstreamed"
(and therefore untreated) throughout their elementary school
years. Despite the belief of well-meaning educators that these
youngsters would derive benefit from being with their peers,
there is no evidence that this occurred. Instead these youngsters emerged from mainstreaming functionally retarded.
They are, at this time, the subjects of an intense remedial
educational program.

More recently I have encountered two previously unidentified schizophrenics who I believe to be suffering from childhood schizophrenia: These young adults somehow made it
through the educational system, and indeed through childhood and most of adolescence without being identified (both
were seen during the adolescent years, although the severity
of their psychopathology was not recognized). Neither of
them was able to function after leaving school. Both have
moderate to severe motor and cognitive deficits in functioning. Both are very immature and affectively constricted, and
both totally lack age-appropriate social and work skills:

Case 1. J.L. was a 24-year-old male who had left school at the age
of 16 having completed ninth grade. At 20 years of age he was
hospitalized, diagnosed as schizophrenic, and placed on major
tranquilizers. At the time when I first saw him he lived with his
mother and left their apartment unaccompanied only to go to
the neighborhood library. He had no friends and had never been
employed.

Case 2. L.B. was a 22-year-old female who presented with very
high anxiety, sleep disturbance, paranoid ideation, total social
isolation, and a history of multiple job failures. This young
woman had a twelfth-grade "business certificate" from a vocational high school. At the time when I first saw her she lived

with her parents and spent her days constantly finding jobs and leaving them just as quickly: She was either fired for irritability and incompetance or she left because she "hated the place."

Are there cases in which childhood schizophrenia spontaneously remits? This question is not answerable with retrospective data. Those cases in which spontaneous remission occurred would be lost to psychiatric follow-up. I have seen a number of children whose families refused treatment. In those cases in which I have some knowledge of follow-up the children were subsequently reidentified by other mental health professionals, as they continued to experience difficulty both educationally and interpersonally.

When developmental disturbance has been minimal in a schizophrenic child, I have recommended mainstreaming. Several of these youngsters have been followed by me, although in some cases years have passed with no psychiatric intervention. In all but one case the fragmented thought process and social ineptness so characteristic of schizophrenia has resulted in the youngster being identified by his or her peers as "odd" or "crazy." A degree of social isolation has been the inevitable outcome. At best these youngsters have been described by the unsophisticated as "weird."

HETEROGENEITY OF THE CHILDHOOD SCHIZOPHRENIC POPULATION

Group 1 versus Group 2

There are profound differences between schizophrenic children. Some of these differences have already been described, as our cohort of 54 childhood schizophrenics appeared to divide itself into two populations, designated by us as Group 1 and Group 2. Prior to observing this "spontaneous" distribution, we had analyzed our data by age of onset, age at time of examination, gender, and clinical subtype (e.g., paranoid, undifferentiated, etc.), all without defining any statistically significant differences.

The distribution of our 54 subjects into Group 1 and Group 2 did reveal statistically significant differences between the two groups that may have some prognostic implications for preschool schizophrenic children. Given the clinical severity of the Group 1 population (Chapters 5 and 6), a preschooler who has a high symptom score relative to his or her physical characteristic score, and who is therefore assigned to Group 1, should be considered a high priority for long-term and intensive treatment services.

Traditional Subtypes

The meaning of encountering the traditional clinical subtypes within the childhood schizophrenic population is less clear. "Pure" paranoids (4 of 25 preschoolers, 3 of 15 latency-aged youngsters, and 5 of 14 adolescents) were uncommon, and "pure" hebephrenics were rare (2 of 25 preschoolers, 0 of 15 latency-aged, and 2 of 14 adolescents). Most often, at least in the early phases of treatment, the children presented a very mixed clinical picture, catatonic posturing and agitation being commonly encountered in association with symptoms of disorganization, disturbances in thought content and process, and affective disturbances.

There is, however, some reason for believing that within the childhood schizophrenic population some clinical presentations may have stability, as paranoid symptomatology has continued to dominate the clinical presentation in the untreated paranoid childhood schizophrenics, and symptoms of disorganization have thus far proven to be quite resistant to both maturation and intensive therapeutic intervention.

There is evidence to suggest that it is particularly dangerous to ignore the paranoid schizophrenic child. Such children may eventually commit murder (Lewis et al., 1985; Schreiber, 1983). I have seen a 6-year-old boy, with a history of paranoid schizophrenia in the immediate family, who was reported to have killed birds with his bare hands. I have seen a young man in his 20s, with a history of "severe emotional disturbance" going back to his childhood, who constantly threatened to harm his mother if he was not "put away." He was left in the community, subsequently severely injured his mother, and is now in a provincial jail. The paranoid children in our treatment programs have been the most resistant to peer-group pressure, and have continued to isolate themselves even in a therapeutic setting. Such children do, however, respond to individual psychotherapy (Cantor & Kestenbaum, 1986). Individual psychotherapy is therefore most urgently recommended. Its effectiveness may, however, be severely limited unless it occurs within the context of a therapeutic milieu such as the one described in the next section.

DESIGNING A THERAPEUTIC MILIEU

The treatment approach that we have found to be effective with very young schizophrenic children has been described elsewhere (Cantor, 1982; Cantor & Kestenbaum, 1986). Helping each child learn how to live with and compensate for the cognitive, sensory, affective, and motor deficits that are so strongly associated with childhood schizophrenic disease provides the unifying focus for this approach to treatment. In this section some details are provided on the mechanics of establishing and operating such a treatment program.

Choosing a Site

Although our treatment approach began in a university teaching hospital, it has been beneficial to relocate to a public elementary school. The school has allowed us the use of a regular classroom setting. Both the staff and the children have benefited from the constant exposure to societal norms. (The importance of such exposure for professionals who are working with disturbed children cannot be overestimated: It is so easy to believe that you have worked a miracle and that a child is now "normal"—if you do not have a normal child around to reality test the staff.) We have been fortunate in that the school also allowed for partial integration: As children have acquired an area of academic strength they have been sent into the regular classroom to cope with that subject.

A school is an optimum place for a treatment program; however, in the event that school placement is not possible it is still desirable to locate within the community as close to a public school as possible. A formal relationship with a nearby elementary school should be negotiated, because partial integration can be of benefit to a psychotic child's educational program.

Alternatively, a private school for severely disturbed children can be therapeutically effective. Such facilities are, unfortunately, very expensive and are therefore not universally accessible.

Hiring a Staff

Treatment programs for psychotic children should be administered by a specially trained physician who accepts the responsibility for administering the program and for establishing treatment priorities. The classroom staff should include a teacher with special expertise in language disorders and a registered psychiatric nurse with a special interest in the psychiatric disorders of childhood. An occupational therapist, with knowledge of the sensory integrative approach to treatment, and a psychotherapist, with a special interest in family therapy with communication-disordered families, should complete the treatment team. Ideally, classroom size should be limited to six preschoolers or eight elementary-aged children.

Establishing Treatment Priorities

Treatment planning for each child should be individualized and ongoing; that is, treatment should begin by determining the child's current level of functioning and outlining short-term interventions based upon that level of functioning. At frequent intervals the child should be reevaluated, and new priorities for treatment should be established.

Our own treatment team has utilized a morning treatment conference for implementing this approach. At these conferences each child is reviewed, on a rotating basis, by the entire treatment team. A card is maintained on each child on which we document the "problems" that are the focus of current interventions.

Within 6 months of admission to treatment, and biannually thereafter, a "strength–deficit evaluation" should be prepared for each child. The child's current functional capacity is described under seven subheadings (Table 18). Completing a strength–deficit assessment on each child greatly facilitates the treatment staff's ability to conceptualize the child's present level of functioning (Figure 19).

The staff's subjective impressions of the child can be augmented by means of formal assessments (e.g., the WISC-R or the B-O) if the child is able to cooperate with testing, and if the team agrees that it requires more objective data in order to make treatment decisions. In addition to providing a profile of current functioning, a biannual strength–deficit evaluation will ensure that at least twice a year the staff will evaluate the effectiveness of its short-term treatment interventions, and that any deterioration in functioning that may be occurring as a result of the progress of the disease will be documented (Figure 19).

An Auxiliary Ego First; Later an Observing and Regulating Ego

There is some agreement that schizophrenia at any age is an ego-deficit syndrome (Freeman, Cameron, & McGhie, 1973). Childhood schizophrenia is not an exception to this general observation. The difficulty schizophrenic children experience with self-regulation is reflected in the Symptom Scale (e.g., "perseveration, poorly regulated anxiety, inappropriate affect, hyperacusis, monotonous vocal inflection, and loose association"; see Chapter 5, Table 15), in measurements of gross and fine motor functioning (see Chapter 6, Table 16), in the elaboration of delusions based upon stories that the child has either heard or read (reflecting a poor ego boundary), and in the persistence of poor posture and abnormal gait (see Chapter 5, Table 14).

The ego controls of children, compared to those of adults, are generally weak (A. Freud, 1965a), and handicapped children as a group are vulnerable to developmental delay (A. Freud, 1965b). At least some of the behavior of schizophrenic children should therefore be understood within the context of normal development. The staff who interact with these children must have a good working knowledge of normal development and must be aware of their own internalized conflicts related to dependence versus autonomy. Symbiotic relationships are all too easily formed with handicapped children. The staff will frequently need to function as an auxiliary ego, but should be sensitive to every attempt the schizophrenic child makes to "do it himself," even when such attempts are sometimes manifest as negative or even paranoid responses.

By 9 or 10 years of age, a schizophrenic child may be capable of forming a therapeutic alliance; that is, the child may be able to recognize the importance of the therapist to the structuring and organizing of experience. The first evidence that this has occurred is often revealed by the child's sudden interest in time, as the day of the week may be defined in relation to the psychotherapy session (Figure 20).

As schizophrenic children mature it will be helpful for them to have a working knowledge of their symptoms. Thus a child who suffers from severe ambivalence may strive for some degree of self-regulation if he or she is encouraged to understand this phenomenon as a "symptom." Such children are often rigid and perfectionistic. Rather than volunteer two conflicting answers to a problem, they frequently remain silent or respond with monosyllables (poverty of speech) while they struggle internally for a definitive answer. They may even stop thinking altogether (thought blocking) if they feel overwhelmed. Similarly children who have no concept of secondary thought process and who verbalize every thought that occurs to them need to be provided with an understanding of the difference between primary and secondary thought process before they can make any voluntary effort to attend to context and to keep themselves on track.

The internalization of self-regulation (i.e., autonomous ego functioning) is the long-term objective of intensive psychotherapy with schizophrenic children. It will, however, be years before the child who has learned to "slow down and think" under the watchful eyes of the treatment team will be able to consistently self-regulate in an unstructured situation (Figures 21 and 22).

Although the child who has begun to develop a self-concept and to self-regulate can be a source of much gratification to the treatment team, the affected child may respond to

Table 18
A strength–deficit approach to treatment

I. Gross motor
 • Describe:
   Gait
   Posture
   The ability to run, climb, and play ball
   The establishment of dominance
   Balance
   Bilateral coordination
   Muscle strength
   Muscle tone
   Motor planning capacity
 • Note the presence of clumsiness if significant; good rhythm if present.
 • Note the presence of gross motor mannerisms; respiratory mannerisms.
II. Fine motor
 • Describe:
   Pincer grasp
   Prehension
   Pencil skills
   Scissor skills
   Draw-a-Person
 • Note fine motor mannerisms
III. Sensorium
 • Describe:
   Observation skills (attention especially)
   Auditory discrimination
   Reaction to being touched
   Visual tracking skills
   Willingness to explore objects with hands
 • Note the presence of primitive or compulsive responses (e.g., mouthing, smelling).
 • Note the presence of hallucinations.
IV. Adaptive
 • Describe:
   Eating behavior
   Dressing behavior (e.g., awareness of sequence)
   Toileting behavior
   Frustration tolerance
   Response to change (e.g., panic, disorganization, etc.)

Table 18
(continued)

Memory skills (e.g., rote only, short-term memory deficits, etc.)
Concept of mastery (i.e., problem-solving skills)
- Note autonomic instability (e.g., easy flushing, pupillary responses, reactive tachycardia).

V. Social
- Describe:
   Ego boundary level
   Affective responses (e.g., constricted, inappropriate)
   Social responsivity (e.g., guarded, friendly)
   Prevailing attitude (e.g., passive, negative, cooperative)
   Prevailing mood (e.g., tearful, labile)
   Play behavior (e.g., perseverative, ability to project, group play)

VI. Language
- Describe:
   Expressive language skills including:
      Use of parts of speech
      Vocabulary
      Grammatical awareness
      Syntax
      Ability to use language to meet needs
      Ability to use language to solicit information
   Language comprehension
- Note the amount of primary process thinking revealed by language (e.g., word salad).
- Note vocal mannerisms, abnormal pitch or tone of voice.

VII. Academics
- Describe:
   Academic strengths and weaknesses using local department of education criteria
   Reading comprehension
   Attitude toward formal learning

---

increasing self-awareness with self-hatred. We have heard children as young as 9 years of age express a wish to die rather than to be different. One child bruised his throat while attempting to "fix" the monotonous voice that had become the brunt of peer-group teasing. The same child burst into a Catholic chapel one day and demanded of God in a loud voice that He immediately make him "normal."

Figure 19

An end-of-the-year strength–deficit assessment of a 5-year-old schizophrenic boy who has just completed a year in our treatment program

I. Gross motor	
Strengths	Deficits

• Dominance established (hand only)
• Fair climber
	• Mixed dominance eye and foot use
	• Poorly coordinated running, walking, and standing
	• Poor endurance
	• Clumsiness
	• Poor:
	    gait
	    balance
	    motor planning
	    postural control
	    control of saliva
	    ballplaying skills
	• Inability to maintain muscle tone (e.g., falls off chairs)
	• Motor mannerisms, including:
	    face slapping
	    breath holding
	    rocking
	    startle response
	    agitation

II. Fine motor	
Strengths	Deficits
• Good prehension • Adequate scissor skills	• Still rakes intermittently • Poor pencil skills (e.g., difficulty reproducing shapes) • Very immature Draw-a-Person • Slight tremor

III. Sensorium	
Strengths	Deficits
• More comfortable with touch	• Increasing preoccupation with internal stimuli • Decreased attention to external stimuli • Slight difficulty with auditory discrimination • Distractable

Figure 19
(continued)

IV. Adaptive

Strengths	Deficits
• Appropriate eating behavior (e.g., serves self, prepares food properly, etc.) • Good dressing skills • Improving self-concept • *Beginning* sense of mastery	• Poor frustration tolerance, although improving • Disorganizes very easily (e.g., in response to stress, change that occurs too rapidly, etc.) • Moderate autonomic instability, (e.g., flushes easily, frequent tachycardia and mydriasis)

V. Social

Strengths	Deficits
• Good motivation and attitude	• Self-perception still very shaky, echopraxia and echolalia at times • Moderate emotional lability

VI. Language

Strengths	Deficits
• Grammatical awareness good • Vocabulary usage appropriate • Parts of speech used appropriately • Syntax good	• Difficulty using language to meet social, cognitive, and emotional needs • Perseverates on "why" • Anxiety consistently interferes with comprehension • Frequent thought intrusions • Occasional psychoticism appears in speech (e.g., clanging, echoing) • Singsong, monotonous voice

VII. Academics

Strengths	Deficits
• Evident facility for mathematics • Has completed academic requirement for kindergarten (i.e., spatial concept, time, size, simple games, puzzle tasks, shapes)	• Difficulty with: sequencing two-step problem solving color discrimination complex stimuli (e.g., Veri-Tech Mosaics)

In sum:
J.B.'s major gain this academic year has been a much improved self-concept; i.e., he now likes himself and believes he can achieve with hard work.

There has, however, been an increase in the symptoms of childhood schizophrenia during the past year; e.g., motor tone has decreased, gross motor functioning has deteriorated, emotional expressivity has decreased (he is less labile), energy level has decreased (he is less hyperactive and more lethargic).

143

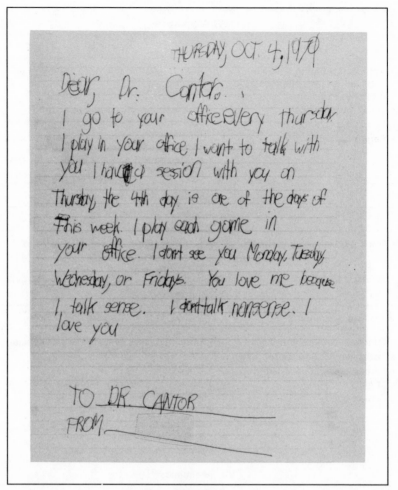

Figure 20
A letter written by a 9-year-old schizophrenic boy to his therapist demonstrating that the child has begun to attend both to concepts of time and to his therapist.

"Why me?" is a painful but natural response to the discovery that one is different. It is difficult to persuade a child who is developmentally handicapped that growing up is not easy for anybody. The child or adolescent with schizophrenia will need time and a private space to work through his or her anger at being different. Given the severity of the motor, language,

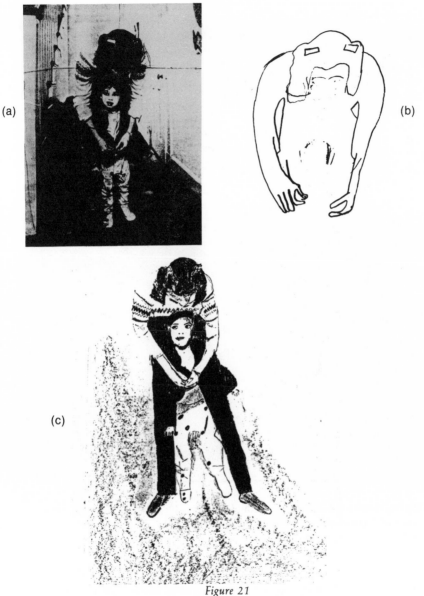

Figure 21

(a) Picture used as class assignment: Each student was to make a freehand copy of it. (b) The first attempts of a 15-year-old schizophrenic boy to complete the assigned freehand drawing. (c) The boy's final copy of the assigned drawing (it was the best in the class) after several days of tracing at the insistence of the treatment staff to help him learn to slow down and observe detail.

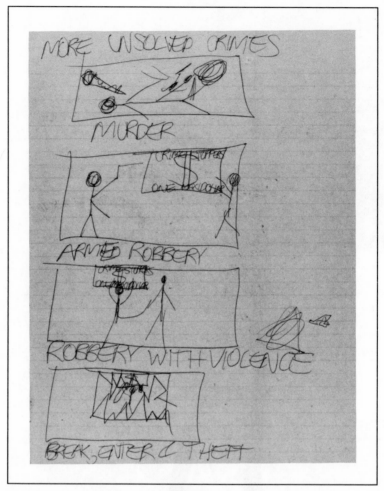

Figure 22

The freehand drawings of the same boy when he is left to his own devices. The stick figures shown here were drawn several weeks after the excellent freehand drawing shown in Figure 21(c).

cognitive, and social deficits associated with this disorder, most childhood schizophrenics will need intensive psychiatric treatment and a supportive network of services throughout their developing years (Cantor, 1982). A healthy concept of self, albeit a damaged self, and a capacity for constructive self-regulation are the hoped-for eventual treatment outcome.

DIAGNOSTIC SCALES

The derivation of the diagnostic scales (Tables 19–21) that should be used to complete the assessment of schizophrenic children has been described in some detail elsewhere (Cantor *et al.*, 1981). As a result of experience with the scales we have made the following modifications:

- "Hyporeflexia" has been deleted in order to facilitate the physical examination (it is difficult to elicit reflexes on a frightened, uncooperative child).
- "True hypercanthism" has been added in order to increase our data base, although it was not a part of the original study and therefore cannot be assigned a weighted score.
- The proviso that the criteria for DSM-III schizophrenia be met has been deleted. DSM-III-R has still made no provision for schizophrenia in children.
- "Dilated pupils" has been deleted as a result of the instability of the sign.
- The radiological sign of decreased muscle mass has been deleted in order to facilitate the use of the scale by physicians without ready access to such services.

CRITERIA FOR SCHIZOPHRENIA, CHILDHOOD TYPE

Five criteria must be met for an individual to be regarded as suffering from childhood schizophrenia (Table 19):

1. A symptom checklist score of at least 9 (raw) and 30 (weighted) must be attained.
2. At least four of the core symptoms should be present.
3. The symptoms must have been present more than 6 months.
4. There must be no known neurological disease present (e.g., posttraumatic head injury, brain tumor, etc.).

Table 19
Criteria for childhood schizophrenia

(meets criteria)

1. _____   1. Symptom checklist score ____ ____
                                                  raw   weighted

2. _____   2. Total number of core symptoms ____

3. _____   3. Symptoms present for more than 6 months

4. _____   4. Known neurological disease ____

5. _____   5. (at least 1 of 3 present)
                         ____ a. Physical Characteristic Scale score

                              ____   ____
                              raw   weighted
                         ____ b. Brunininks–Oseretsky: Mean ____

                              ____ ____

                              ____ ____

                         ____ c. (at least 4 signs present)
                              Lordosis ____
                              Strabismus ____
                              Articular defect ____
                              Flat feet ____
                              Loss of flexor tone ____
                              No arm swing ____
                              Waddling gait ____

---

5. At least one of the following must be satisfied:
   a. Physical Characteristic Scale score of at least 7 (raw) or 18
      (weighted) has been recorded.
   b. The youngster has achieved a standard score of 6 or less
      on at least four subsections of the Bruininks–Oseretsky.
   c. Four of the seven signs of neuromuscular dysfunction are
      present.

SYMPTOM SCALE

The Symptom Scale score sheet (Table 20) is best completed during
one or more unstructured play sessions (prepubertal subjects) or
during an unstructured psychiatric interview (some latency and all
postpubertal subjects). It is recommended that the following guidelines be used in completing the scale:

• The examining psychiatrist should take extensive notes.
  These should include verbatim examples of primary process

thinking, which would otherwise be very difficult to remember (the normal human brain "tunes out" disordered communication).

- "Mannerisms" should be regarded as present only if motor mannerisms other than facial grimacing are noted. Common examples include clicking noises, blowing, breath holding followed by blowing it out, etc.

Table 20
Symptom Scale

	[✓]	Weighted score (circle if present)
Flat or severely constricted affect (excluding anxiety)*	____	5
Perseveration*	____	5
Good eye contact when communicating needs	____	5
Inappropriate affect (episodic giggling or crying)*	____	4
High anxiety (intermittent)	____	4
Fragmentation of thought*	____	4
Hypersensitivity	____	4
Monotonous speech or bradylalia	____	3
Loose association (derailment)*	____	3
Neologisms	____	2
Echolalia or delayed echolalia	____	2
Illogicality*	____	2
Mannerisms (usually noise)	____	2
Grimace*	____	2
Perplexity	____	2
Autism (preoccupation with inner stimuli)	____	2
Clang associations	____	1
Incoherence*	____	1
Raw score	____	
Weighted score		____

Associated symptoms
Poverty of speech ____   Paranoia ____
Poverty of content of speech ____   Delusions ____
Amvibalence ____   Hallucinations ____

Note. Asterisks (*) indicate core symptoms.

Table 21
Physical Characteristic Scale

	[✓]	Weighted score (circle if present)
Hypotonia	___	5
Brachycephaly $\left[\dfrac{\text{Lat.}}{\text{A-P}} \geq 0.8\right]$[a]	___	4
Long hands (>75%)	___	4
Decreased muscle power	___	4
Decreased muscle mass	___	3
Blue eyes	___	3
Hypercanthism (>75%)	___	2
True hypercanthism (>97%)	___	
Soft velvety skin	___	2
Head > height	___	2
Increased head circumference (>75%)	___	1
Prominent nasal bridge	___	1
Deep-set eyes	___	1
Short fingers $\left[\dfrac{\text{MF}}{\text{HL}} \leq 25\%\right]$[b]	___	1
Lax elbows	___	1
Lax MCP joints and wrists	___	1
Raw score	___	
Weighted score		___

[a]Lat., lateral diameter; A-P, anterior–posterior diameter.
[b]MF, middle finger; HL, hand length.

- "Perplexity" in a very young child is usually revealed by a puzzled frown; schizophrenic children seldom indicate their puzzlement verbally.
- "Autism" may be revealed by self-referential statements or by a constant attention to inner drives and stimuli (much more difficult to score with certainty in a prepubertal child).
- "Incoherence" is scored only if the child is clearly trying to communicate and the communication is incomprehensible (e.g., this sign was usually observed as self-talk during the projective play of schizophrenic children).

PHYSICAL CHARACTERISTIC SCALE

The Physical Characteristic Scale (Table 21) must be used in conjunction with normative data (provided in Figure 24 for three characteristics). The following guidelines should be followed in using the scale:

- "Hypotonia" should be scored if the child's limbs respond floppily to passive movement (i.e., the child does not maintain normal resting tone), if the child cannot maintain active resistance to being manipulated (and most frightened children will certainly struggle to maintain such resistance), and if no muscle mass can be palpated in the resting limb (i.e., the muscle feels "doughy"). The presence of the "associated signs" should reassure the physician who is concerned with the subjectivity of this sign.
- "Brachycephaly" is scored by utilizing an obstetrical caliper to measure the greatest lateral diameter (Figure 23a) and the greatest anterior–posterior (A-P) diameter (Figure 23b). The ratio of the lateral to the A-P diameter is normally 0.7 to 0.8. A ratio greater than 0.8 is termed brachycephaly; one less than 0.7 is termed dolichocephaly.
- "Decreased muscle power" is a totally subjective measure. If the child tries to resist the examiner and quickly loses voluntary muscle power, it can be assumed that decreased muscle power is present.
- "Decreased muscle mass" should be scored only if the child or adolescent lack normal muscle contour (see Chapter 4).
- "Hypercanthism" should be measured as indicated in Figure 23c. (Normative data are shown graphically in Figure 24a.)
- "Soft velvety skin" should be assessed over the abdomen, since clothing normally roughens the abdominal surface.
- Both "prominent nasal bridge" and "deep-set eyes" are assessed by viewing the subject in profile. Both of these signs should be quite marked to be scored as present.
- "Short fingers" are assessed by measuring the ratio of middle finger length (Figure 23e) to hand length (Figure 23d). This ratio is age dependent, and normative data are therefore provided (see Figure 24, b and c).
- "Lax joints" are assessed by determining the automatic resistance encountered to passive movement (the child is told to relax; most children don't relax, but hyperextension is nevertheless observed).

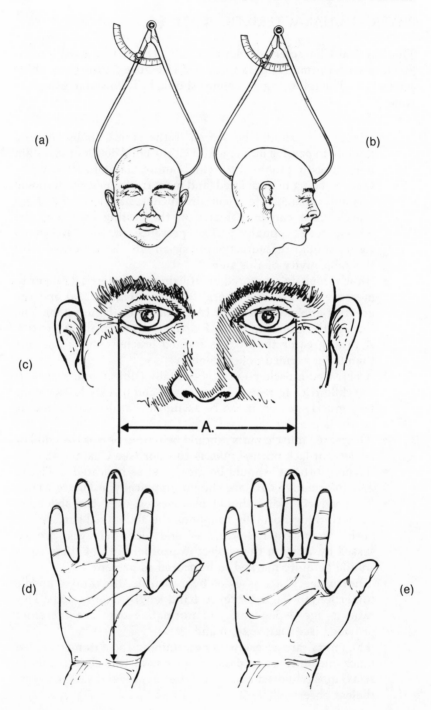

The associated physical signs (see Chapter 5 and Table 19, Criterion 5c) should be recorded as unobtrusively as possible; for example, one can observe the child walking to and from one's office. The most difficult sign to assess is "strabismus" because, in many children, this is no longer obvious by the time of psychiatric assessment. The only sign of strabismus that may still persist is an abnormal light reflex (the light reflex on the two eyes should be symmetrical).

Figure 23
(a–e) Figures illustrating the exact positioning of the tape measure or calipers to be used by the physician during the assessment of the physical characteristics. Measures for brachycephaly: (a) lateral diameter; (b) anterior–posterior diameter. (c) Measure for outer canthal distance. Measures for short fingers: (d) hand length; (e) middle finger length.

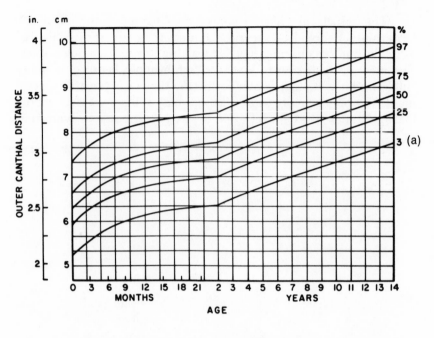

(a)

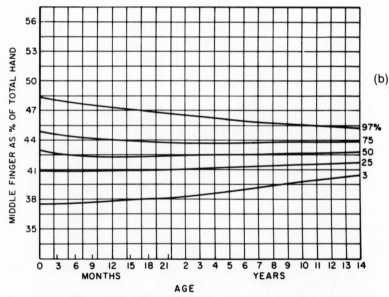

(b)

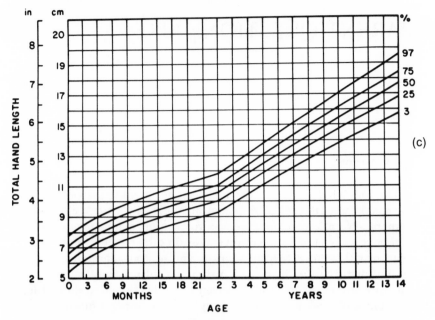

Figure 24

Graphs of normative data on age-dependent characteristics. (a) Outer can-
thal distance. (b) Middle finger/hand length ratio. (c) Total hand length.
From Feingold, M., & Bossert, W. H. "Normal Values for Selected Physical
Parameters: An Aid to Syndrome Delineation," in D. Bergsma (Ed.), *Birth
Defects: Original Articles Series* (Vol. 10, p. 13). White Plains, NY: National
Foundation-March of Dimes, 1974. Reprinted with permission.

PARENT QUESTIONNAIRE

Dear Parents:

The following questionnaire has been designed to provide us with the maximum amount of information regarding your child's development. We ask your forgiveness for asking many questions that you have answered several times over on different occasions. However, it will be most helpful to us in coming to understand developmental disturbances if we can gather the information requested in this questionnaire from all children with developmental disorders. Therefore, we ask your cooperation in filling out this questionnaire.

If your child is less than 5 years old, answer the parts of the questionnaire that pertain to your child's age group (i.e., omit the section having to do with ages 5–6). Do not hesitate to leave unanswered questions about which you have doubts. We ask your forgiveness if remembering your child's difficulties with development causes pain.

Please provide your answers in the spaces provided. If the question is a yes–no type, please put the number "1" in the space to indicate "yes" and the number "2" in the space to indicate "no." If the question is "not applicable," please place the number "3" in the space provided.

PART I. FAMILY INFORMATION

	First name	Birthdate	Occupation	Highest education achieved
1. Father	_____	___ ___ ___	_____	_____
2. Mother	_____	___ ___ ___	_____	_____

3. When married _____

4. Related before marriage? _____

5. Child's siblings: Number _____

6. Child's birth position (i.e., 1st, 2nd, etc.) _____

7. Brothers and sisters (in order, including miscarriages or still-births)

First name	Date of birth	Present occupation (e.g., grade in school, job)

8. List below any family members who have suffered from any of the following (include only brothers and sisters of the child named herein, grandparents, uncles, and aunts). Give details; state relationship of affected relative and nature of disorder (e.g., mongolism).

Mental retardation   _____

Learning disability   _____

Speech delay   _____

Epilepsy   _____

Mental illness   _____

Suicide   _____

Alcoholism   _____

PART II. PREGNANCY

1. Did you have an intrauterine device in place when you became pregnant? _____

2. Were you on the birth control pill when you became pregnant? _____

3. Did you take any medication during the pregnancy? _____

4. Medication	Amount (dosage)	Trimester taken:		
		1st	2nd	3rd
Aspirin _____	_____	_____	_____	_____
Antibiotics _____	_____	_____	_____	_____
Sleeping pills _____	_____	_____	_____	_____

Valium and related drugs
(specify)

_____   _____   ___   ___   ___

_____   _____   ___   ___   ___

Other (include any other
over-the-counter
preparation)

_____   _____   ___   ___   ___

_____   _____   ___   ___   ___

5. Did you smoke cigarettes during the pregnancy? ____
   Number of cigarettes per day (on average)
      1st trimester ____
      2nd trimester ____
      3rd trimester ____

6. Did you drink alcoholic beverages during the pregnancy? ____
   Amount* per day (on average)
      1st trimester ____
      2nd trimester ____
      3rd trimester ____
   *1 = 1 oz of hard liquor or 1 beer or 4 oz wine.

7. Did you obtain prenatal care? ____

8. Did you experience any of the following during the pregnancy?

	Trimester:		
	1st	2nd	3rd
Vomiting	___	___	___
Bleeding or spotting	___	___	___
Excessive swelling (of hands or feet)	___	___	___
Sugar in urine	___	___	___
Infectious episode (include all illnesses, even minor viral)	___	___	___
High blood pressure	___	___	___

Were you hospitalized for any reason during the
   pregnancy? ____
   If so, describe _____

_____

9. Do you suffer from any of the following?
   Diabetes   ____
   Kidney disease   ____
   Chronic illness for which you take medication   ____

PART III. LABOR AND DELIVERY

1. Labor began:
   At term   ____
   Before term: ____ weeks
   After term: ____ weeks

2. Onset of labor was signaled by:
   "Show"   ____
   Water breaking   ____
   Contractions   ____

3. Hospital of delivery   _____
   Address of hospital   _____
   Attending physician   _____

4. Length of labor, in hours   ____

5. Was any means used to hasten labor?
   Intravenous drip   ____
   Breaking water   ____

6. Were you asleep when the baby was born?   ____

7. Was delivery:
   Vaginal?   ____
   Cesarean?   ____

8. When you first saw the baby, was the head normal in
   shape?   ____

9. Were there any difficulties during the delivery?
   Cord around the neck   ____
   Delay in breathing   ____
   Other (specify)   _____

10. Birthweight: _____ _____
                    lb   oz

11. Course in hospital (describe how the baby did in the first few days of life and whether there were any complications)

    _____

    _____

    _____

12. Complications _____
    No complications _____

13. Was the baby born with any deformities?
    Large birthmark _____
    Heart defect _____
    Inguinal hernia _____
    Club feet _____
    Other (specify) _____

    _____

PART IV. EARLY INFANCY

1. Feeding:
   How did you feed the baby?
      Breast _____
      Formula _____
   Comment on any difficulties, etc. _____

   _____

   Was suck strong and did the baby eat well? _____
   Was the baby colicky? _____

2. Sleep:
   Was the baby a light _____ or heavy _____ sleeper?
   Did the baby sleep between feedings? _____
   Was the baby contented _____ or irritable _____?
   When the baby was awake, was he or she alert _____
   or lethargic _____?

PART V. THE FIRST YEAR

1. Were there any major illnesses during the first year of life? _____
   If so, list _____

   _____

2. Any operations or hospitalizations? _____
   If so, specify _____

3. When did the baby first:
   Smile ___ weeks
   Hold head ___ weeks
   Sit unsupported ___ months
   Stand unsupported ___ months
   Take first step ___ months
   Move about independently ___ months
   Imitate your sounds (e.g., "mama") ___ months

4. Did the baby like to be picked up? ___

5. Did the baby anticipate being picked up (e.g., look up in anticipation or hold up arms)? ___

6. Did the baby sleep:
   In a curled up position? ___
   With limbs outstretched? ___

7. Did the baby babble? ___

8. Did the baby show an interest in his or her environment? ___

9. Did the baby demonstrate any repetitive movement?
   Rocking ___
   Head banging ___
   Other (specify) _____

10. Did the baby welcome your company? ___

11. Was the baby unusually fearful (e.g., cry at loud noises or strangers, etc.)? ___

12. Did the baby differentiate between major caretakers (such as mother and father) and strangers? ___

13. How old was the baby when he or she first differentiated between caretakers and strangers? ___

14. Did the baby have an "unusual" attitude toward people? ____
    If so, describe _____

_____

15. Did the baby use a sucking object?
    Thumb ____
    Fingers ____
    Blankets ____
    Other (specify) _____

_____

16. Did the baby take well to solid foods? ____
    If no, describe problem _____

_____

17. Did the baby have crib playthings? ____

18. How did the baby react to crib playthings?
    Ignored them ____
    Played only when adult initiated ____
    Played independently with them ____
    Was fearful of them ____
    Other (specify) _____

_____

19. Was the baby a curious infant (e.g., reach for objects to see how
    they worked, roll and crawl to interesting objects in order to
    investigate them, etc.)? ____

PART VI. AGES 1–4 YEARS

1. How did your child communicate between ages 1 and 2 (check all
   applicable)?
   Gestures ____
   Take your hand and pull you ____
   Verbalization ____
   Other (specify _____

_____

2. As your child grew older, did he or she get more and more
   curious? ____

3. Note the age at which your child was able to relate in the manner described (if not at all, answer NA):

Relate with:	To meet basic needs	Age	Comfort seeking	Age	Relaxed play	Age
Major caretakers (e.g., parents)	___	___	___	___	___	___
Adult friends and acquaintances	___	___	___	___	___	___
Strangers	___	___	___	___	___	___
Older children	___	___	___	___	___	___
Peer children	___	___	___	___	___	___

4. Did your child like toys? ___

5. At ages 1–4 which types of toys did your child like?

		Favorite?
Vehicles	___	___
Blocks	___	___
Puzzles	___	___
Fantasy	___	___
Dolls, house	___	___

6. (a) Did your child play with toys according to their function, such as roll a car, build with blocks; or (b) did your child use all toys in the same way, for example, bang everything?
   (a) ___   (b) ___

7. Did your child choose a favorite object to carry around and to take to bed (such as a teddy bear, other stuffed animals, a blanket, etc.)? ___
   If so, specify _____
   _____

8. Were there any occurrences or objects that especially troubled your child (such as loud noises, clothes with rough material, etc.)? ___
   If so, specify _____
   _____

9. Did you child avoid any special toys or objects (e.g, rocking horses, slides, swings, etc.)? ___
   If so, specify _____
   _____

10. Indicate the age at which the following first occurred:
Eye contact ____ months
Gesturing to get attention ____ months
Verbal imitation ____ months
Attempted verbalization (i.e., jibberish) ____ months
Word usage ____ months
Sentence usage ____ months
Comments: _____

11. Major illnesses or hospitalizations during this period (ages 1–4)? ____

Illness	Age (in months)	Course of illness
_____	___	_____
_____	___	_____

12. Did your child suffer from any high fevers during this time? ____

	Age (in months)	Cause if known
_____	___	_____
_____	___	_____

13. When (in months) did your child first attempt to climb stairs? ____

14. How old was your child (in months) before he or she was able to take the stairs in sequence instead of one at a time? ____
Up ____
Down ____

15. Did your child develop any unusual behaviors during this time?
Rocking ____
Heading banging ____
Biting or scratching self ____
Continuing to put all objects in mouth after age 18 months ____
Other (specify) _____

16. Was there anything unusual about the way your child walked?
Toe walking ____
Waddling ____
Other (specify) _____

17. How did your child usually react to frustration?
    Temper tantrums ____
       Describe _____
    _____

    Withdrawal ____
       Describe _____
    _____

    Other (specify and describe) _____
    _____

18. Did your child have any difficulty falling asleep?
    12–24 months ____
    24–36 months ____
    36–48 months ____

19. Did your child usually sleep through the night?
    12–24 months ____
    24–36 months ____
    36–48 months ____

20. Did your child usually wake for the day before 6 A.M.?
    12–24 months ____
    24–36 months ____
    36–48 months ____

21. When did toilet training begin (in months)? ____

22. When was toilet training accomplished (in months)? ____

23. How was toilet training accomplished? _____
    _____

24. How did your child typically spend the waking hours (choose all
    applicable behaviors) between ages 2 and 4?

    Inactive, aimless behavior ____
    Sedentary, playing alone ____
    Sedentary, playing with someone ____
    Active, playing alone ____
    Active, playing with someone ____
    Other (specify) _____
    _____

25. Describe *preferred* behavior in some detail: _____

_____

_____

PART VII. AGES 5–6 YEARS

1. At what age did your child begin school? ___ years, ___ months

2. What was the first school your child attended?
   Name _____
   Address _____

3. Describe your child's first reaction to school.
   Liked ___
   Disliked ___
   Unaffected by experience ___
   Fearful ___
   Elaborate: _____

   _____

4. Did the reaction change? ___

5. If so, after how many months of school? ___

6. Describe any events related to or sources of the change as you
   understand them: _____

   _____

7. If your child had *no* difficulties prior to beginning school, describe
   what difficulties were encountered in school, when they were
   encountered, and what was recommended.

		Age of child (in years and months)	Recommendations
Social difficulties	___	___, ___	_____
Emotional difficulties	___	___, ___	_____
Academic difficulties	___	___, ___	_____
Other (specify)	___	___, ___	_____
_____	___	___, ___	_____

   Elaborate (i.e., outcome of problem): _____

   _____

8. Did your child like toys at this age? ____

9. What type(s) of toys did your child like?

                                           Favorite?
   Vehicles   ____   ____
   Blocks   ____   ____
   Puzzles   ____   ____
   Fantasy (house, doll)   ____   ____

10. Did your child play with toys appropriately (i.e., ride bike, color in coloring books, etc.)? ____
    Elaborate: _____

    _____

11. Did your child play with other children? ____

12. How would you describe your child's typical interaction with other children at this age?
    Disinterest ____
    Curiosity ____
    Submissive ____
    Dominance ____
    Cooperativeness ____
    Open hostility ____
    Other (specify) _____

    _____

13. Did your child have any difficulties in playing with *more than one* other child at a time? ____

14. Did your child relate well to adults? ____
    Elaborate: _____

    _____

15. Did your child have any unusual fears? ____
    Elaborate: _____

    _____

16. Did your child have any eating problems at this time? ____
    Ate too much ____
    Difficulty eating enough ____
    Unusual food preferences ____
    Specific foods avoided to an unusual degree ____

Other (specify) _____

  Elaborate: _____

  _____

17. Did your child have any difficulties with sleep at this age?
    Slept too much (more than 12 hours) ___
    Slept at unusual hours ___
    Trouble falling asleep ___
    Fitful sleep and/or wakings during night ___
    Early wakings in morning without going back to sleep
      (before 6 A.M.) ___
    Other (specify) _____

    _____

18. List any illnesses or operations that occurred during this time
    period.

                                              Age (in years and months)

    _____   ___, ___

    _____   ___, ___

19. Describe course of each illness.

    _____

    _____

20. Add any information that you feel may be helpful concerning
    this period of your child's life.

    _____

    _____

PART VIII. ADDITIONAL INFORMATION
REGARDING SPEECH

1. Did your child ever reverse pronouns (such as say "you" when
   he or she meant "I")? ___

2. If so, is the problem resolved now? ___

3. Does (or did) your child speak in sentences rather than three- or
   four-word phrases by age 4? ___

4. If no, at what age did your child begin to speak sentences?

——, ——
years months

5. Still doesn't. ——

6. Does (or did) your child make up words that you cannot understand? ——

7. Does (or did) your child ever have other problems with grammar (such as reversing subjects and nouns, etc.)? ——

8. If yes, specify _____

_____

9. Does (or did) your child receive speech therapy? ——

10. If yes, give details (i.e., with whom, when, and where) ——

_____

PART IX. DEVELOPMENTAL CONCERNS

1. When did you first become concerned about your child's development? (age of child, in months) ——

2. What was your first concern about your child?

_____

_____

3. What were other concerns as they developed?

When developed
(age, in months)

_____ ——

_____ ——

4. Whom did you first consult, and when?

When consulted
(age of child,
Name *in months)*

Family physician _____ ——
Child guidance _____ ——
Other (specify) _____ ——

5. What were you told at that time (and by whom)? _____

_____

6. Add anything else you think is relevant (i.e., if your child began school during this age period describe your experience and the reaction of the teachers).

_____

_____

HISTORICAL NOTES

A1. M. Brierre de Boismont (1857): "We found it would be dangerous to keep such a patient; he therefore returned home and we lost sight of him" [the child had been violent, had threatened to set fires and to kill if he could "find a knife"] (p. 624).

"His instincts became more and more perverted, and as he uttered threats perpetually, would strike and try to wound, and talked continually of killing some one, his mother determined to bring him to the asylum. There he became the terror and scourge of the patients, always pinching, biting and striking" (p. 624).

". . . perversions of instinct, of sentiment, and of the moral faculties, rather than well-defined types of mania or monomania" (p. 625).

A2. J. Conolly (1861–1862): "Cases of the kind are rarely met with in Asylums, nor are they, indeed, very common in private practice; but they are not now disregarded or overlooked as they appear to have been. In all probability they were formerly looked upon as instances of perverseness or wickedness, and the unfortunate children were merely chastised, with little advantage" (p. 395).

"In innumerable respects society and manners and modes of thinking have undergone great changes since the beginning of this century, but in no respect more strikingly than in the greater attention paid to the minds of children of every class; as if it had only now been found out that the mind was an attribute of value in every human being" (p. 396).

Conolly points out that mentally handicapped children have "all attracted special attention" and that the "remarkable improvement found to be attainable in a great proportion of them, although a perfect cure is not to be expected, seems to have had a sensible effect in inducing parents . . . to seek advice . . . [while acknowledging that] the uneasiness of parents seldom leads them to seek advice on the subject of their children, however eccentric, untill their gradually increasing strength and independence make their eccentricities inconvenient. . . . Even then, the solicitude for the character and progress of unmanageable children is yet chiefly confined to families of the educated portion of the community" (pp. 396 and 397).

A3. Conolly's clinical descriptions of disturbed children were remarkably detailed. These included:

a. Behavioral observations: "absence of affection . . . indifferent to their parents . . . unmoved by praise or blame . . . fond of inflicting pain on younger children . . . the attention is vaguely shifted from one object to the other . . . affection, giving place when the child is urged to do the slightest thing at variance with its humor, to a frantic expression, and a paroxysmal violence, in which it throws itself down, screams, kicks, and loses all sense of any danger to which its furious actions expose it" (pp. 398-399).

b. Descriptions of posture: "the head is not carried erectly, the trunk is drooping" (p. 397).

c. Descriptions of motility disorders: "there is continual movement of the hands . . . there is a disposition to be always moving from place to place sometimes with a mischievous object, and sometimes with none that can be understood" (p. 397).

d. Observations on physiognomy: "there is generally something peculiar in the shape of the head" (p. 397).

A4. "The physician has a boy presented to his notice, eleven or twelve years of age, tall, pale, delicate-looking; the forehead rather narrow, the occiput rather large, the countenance placid, the speech perfect, and whose replies are quite rational: the manner of the boy, however has a careless and indifferent, character more easy to observe than to describe. . . . He is, however, fond of reading anything in rhyme, little poems, and songs, and hymns. For prose he has small inclination. He is fond of music, and is learning already to play on some instrument. He has no distaste for some kinds of application, even for application to arithmetic. He takes some pleasure in regarding the operations of workmen, and has some especial satisfaction in watching the execution of various kinds of carpenter's work. But notwithstanding this, his most particular inclination is to do nothing. . . . and he has sometimes expressed it to be his early-formed conviction that the pleasures of refined life were constraining and irksome, and, in his estimation, not to be compared with the quiet enjoyment of idleness, and of malt liquor, and of smoking. He shows no absolutely vicious tendencies, and is inoffensive if not thwarted; but if thwarted he is passionate and abusive" (Conolly, 1861-1862, p. 400).

A5. "Both history and the experience of any observant man will furnish examples of very unmanageable boys becoming valuable and even distinguished men" (Conolly, 1861-1862, p. 398).

A6. "The general treatment both in boys and girls comprises the whole range of physical and moral training; and although many boys, more or less deranged . . . may . . . with the advantage of proper care, grow up into useful and good men, many more are ruined for want of it" (Conolly, 1861–1862, p. 403).

Conolly did, however, recognize the difficulty of involving patients in appropriate treatment: "No very satisfactory or continued observation can be generally made of the course of juvenile insanity. Advice is rather reluctantly sought, and is seldom carefully followed; and the proceedings afterwards are seldom accurately reported, or the true history known, even in the case of boys. When girls are the subjects of the malady, still greater care is taken to conceal it, sometimes with little regard for the consequences to those who may become their husbands" (p. 402).

A7. H. Maudsley (1880): "There are boys who, being somewhat stupid and of melancholy, moody, and perhaps morose disposition, habitually keep apart from their fellows, whom they join not in play. They are often hypochondriacal, complaining of strange morbid sensations in abdomen, generative organs, heart or head; and when these morbid feelings are very active they become paroxysmally excited so as to quite lose self-control, and perhaps imagine that the devil has got hold of them. Or some other foolish or insane idea or impulse springs up in the apt soil of their affective perversions and instigates them to foolish or insane conduct. When they reach puberty they show more insanity and perhaps get into trouble . . ." (p. 278).

A8. "In the insanity of the young child we meet with passion in all its naked deformity and in all its exaggerated exhibition. . . . Haslam reports a case of this kind in a girl, aged three and a quarter years, who had become mad at two and a half years of age, after inoculation for small-pox. Her mother's brother was, however, an idiot, though her parents were sane and undiseased. This creature struggled to get hold of everything which she saw, and cried, bit, and kicked if she was disappointed. Her appetite was voracious, and she would devour any sort of food without discrimination; she would rake out the fire with her fingers, and seemed to forget that she had been burnt; she passed her evacuations anywhere. She could not be taught anything, and never improved" (Maudsley, 1880, pp. 282–283).

A9. Maudsley cites another case: "Haslam relates the following case of a young gentleman, aged ten, in whose ancestors no insanity was acknowledged. When only two years old, he was so mischievous and uncontrollable that he was sent from home; and until he was nine years old he continued 'the creature of volition and the terror of the family' and was indulged in every way: he tore his clothes, broke whatever he could break, and often would not take his food. Severe discipline was tried, but in vain; and the boy was ultimately sent to a lunatic asylum. There was deficient sensibility of the skin. He had a very retentive memory with regard to matters which he had witnessed, but was attracted only by fits and starts, so that he could not learn methodically: he was 'the hopeless pupil of many masters,' breaking windows, crockery, and anything else which he could break. . . . He was quite insensible to kindness and never played with other boys. 'Of his own disorder he was sometimes sensible: he would often express a wish to die, for he said very truly, 'God had not made him like other children;' and when provoked he would threaten to destroy himself. No improvement took place" (p. 286).

A10. H. Goddard (1920): "The children are usually more or less solitary; they do not get along well with other children of the same mental level. . . . They are apt to prefer adults to people of their own age. Their games may have a queer monotony which makes them seem peculiar even in their own family. . . . They are apt to have violent tempers and have often been recognized as different from the time they were babies" (p. 515).

A11. "As to the prognosis and treatment of the general run of psychopathic cases still less is known. Some . . . seem to get well; the natural growth processes apparently overcoming to a large extent, if not completely, any effect of the disturbing factor. So that while these cases may show the marks of the disease to the expert, nevertheless the condition does not so far interfere with life as to make them distinctly abnormal personalities. . . . Apparently another group remains unchanged and the victims grow up to be nervous, unstable men and women, easily becoming delinquents and antisocial members of the community. . . . A third group grows progressively worse and finally distinctly insane and contributes to the adult insane population" (Goddard, 1920, p. 516).

A12. L. Witmer (1920): "I saw Donald for the first time when he was 2 years and 7 months old. His father carried him into my office and deposited him, a soulless lump, upon the couch. He sat there . . . absorbed in the inspection of a card which he held in his pudgy hands, as regardless of his father and mother as of the new objects about him. While his gaze moved over the card, he scratched the back of it gently and incessantly with his finger nails. At times he gritted his teeth; and then again he made a crooning, humming sound with which it is his habit to lull himself to sleep. . . . every effort to remove the card from his hands he resisted. His face, already crimson, became empurpled. . . . In the months to come I was to discover that by preference he would sit or lie in bed for hours, looking attentively at the object which he happened to be holding in his hands" (p. 98).

A13. W. C. Hulse (1954; translation of Heller's 1930 report): ". . . [A girl] who began to show peculiarities at age 5, laughing occasionally without reason, whispering to herself words which made no sense. Later she showed a preference for odd positions, appeared sometimes as though 'rooted to the spot,' would get stuck occasionally in the middle of an action, for instance, raising her hand with a spoon without getting it into her mouth. . . . She ran away from her nurse during outdoor walks. She lost interest in games, became whining, negativistic, incontinent. At the age of seven, one could not induce her to get up; she stayed in bed and had to be spoon-fed, taking little nourishment, often for several days. She lost control over urine and feces and remained lying in this dirty mess. . . . was admitted to my institution. . . . The child was first catatonic with outspoken flexibilitas cerea. Occasionally, this catatonic state was interrupted by a state of excitement. In this state, the child would run around, touch everything, throw things to the floor as if in a state of high spirits. Everything edible was consumed ravenously. . . . She spoke Polish and German words in a disconnected way. She carried out orders; on occasions she even did some sewing or other little housework during such a period showing remarkable manual dexterity. Then suddenly and unexpectedly the catatonic state returned . . . but one had the impression that even in the catatonic state, S. observed whatever was going on around her. . . . when once again, she moved freely about the room, she found without hesitation things in the closet which the nurse had put there while the child had been lying in bed. . . . step by step, the child's intelligence declined more and more. She stopped speaking, became unable to keep herself occupied in the simplest fashion, and was unable to understand the meaning and use of the tools and toys put at her disposal. The catatonia moved into the background more and more and was replaced by a state of silliness and idiotic regression" (p. 476).

A14. A. Childers (1931): "Problem as referred: 'patient swears and uses filthy language; "queer" conduct rather than wrong conduct. No interest in school work. Wastes time of whole class.' When he was eight, four and half years ago, a note recorded at school is as follows: 'At times he disturbs by destroying the seat work of children sitting near. He talks to himself and annoys others. Is very nervous, cannot sit still.'"

"Walking and talking were somewhat delayed. The mother states that he would run away as soon as he learned to walk, so that she placed a tag on him with his name and address. . . . He has long had a habit of touching everything he sees. . . . He talks a good deal in his sleep. . . . His mother kept him at home for six months because the teachers wanted him to repeat kindergarten. She blamed the teachers, claiming that they did not teach him proper school habits. He failed twice from lack of effort. . . . Teachers often reported that it was his conduct which held him back; he talked so much. One teacher, who noticed that he did not associate much with other children, asked a boy to walk to school with him each day. This boy tried it once, but reported that the patient insisted upon ringing the doorbells of each house. . . . Little 'wild' tricks of this sort made the children quite intolerant of him. In class, he would suddenly laugh aloud for no apparent reason. . . ." (pp. 121–122).

"He told about his tempers with other children as if he were in no way to blame and other children should accept his conduct. . . . 'They call me "Goofy" and "Nutsy." ' . . . They pick on me all the time just because I don't do their way. They made me go up and ring doorbells when I didn't want to.' . . . He went on to blame his teachers for his poor work in school, saying that they had it in for him and none had ever liked him. . . . He had a very long account of the 'haunts' which have visited him both in his dreams and when awake. 'Some kind of fingers were pinching me in the neck and it seemed they were trying to get me.' He described the 'haunt' variously as, for instance, something like a 'shadow stamping on the roof.' . . . 'All of this has made me have funny feelings in my body.' . . . 'It seemed like a spoon and a dishpan were talking out loud to me.' . . . 'One night I saw lights being switched on, and the 'haunt' came by, and something made me raise my hands up. It's funny it never touched my father, and he didn't believe it happened'" (pp. 122–123).

A15. "We have here a very poorly adjusted boy, to say the least. His phantasies seem to have developed to the degree of actual psychotic experiences at times. . . . The material that he has given regarding strange influences and bodily changes might easily be produced by adult schizophrenic cases. . . . In many respects he has to start now at twelve to learn things that other boys learn many years earlier. . . . he has not at all given up the struggle for adjustment, and he has some favorable interests and drives that can be utilized in reconstruction" (Childers, 1931, pp. 124–125).

A16. H. Potter (1933): "In discussing schizophrenia in children, it is important to give consideration to the facilities which children possess for expressing any form of psychopathology. . . . It must be remembered that the level of intellectual development and the life experiences of the child are limited in comparison with those of the adult. . . . Children are essentially beings of feeling and behavior. Consequently, their psychopathology may be expected to be expressed largely through distorted affective responses and altered behavior reactions" (pp. 1253–1254).

A17. A portion of a case history reads: "During the six months' period during which he has been under observation in the institute, silly laughter, grimacing, and blinking have continued throughout. On many occasions he has been observed to attitudinize with arms partially raised in the air or held at an angle away from the side of the body. At other times he is observed making stereotyped writing motions in the air. He usually carries his head, chin tilted, upward and partially to one side. He will obey commands automatically. He never makes any attempt to integrate himself with the group of children on the ward. He attends school class, does 2B grade work satisfactorily with some individual attention. School work, singing and dancing games in the gymnasium are the only activities thus far which secure his indifferent attention. He will read in a monotonous undertone in an automatic fashion when asked by the teacher. He sings softly to himself and laughs to himself frequently in school class. He is indifferent to his family's visits. He seldom makes adequate reply to questions and to most questions he replies in a high pitched and subdued tone of voice with a far off expression, with a stereotyped 'sombody', 'sometime', 'somewhere'. His affective tone is one of indifferent disinterest and preoccupation" (Potter, 1933, pp. 1258–1259).

A18. Kasanin and Veo (1932): "In the first group (Group I) we have 12 children of unusually striking personality, in the sense that everybody in the school noticed that these children were odd, peculiar and queer. . . . They were often called 'crazy' by other pupils. . . . Here we have the cases that were obviously psychotic but went on for years without showing much change until something dramatic developed which brought the children to the mental hospital. . . . they always gave the teachers the feeling that something dreadful might eventually happen to them" (p. 215).

A case study illustrates a member of Group I: "The principal of the school remembered the patient well, as a very peculiar child. She was extremely unresponsive, and when he made an announcement that was pleasing to the other children, she would sit without any expression on her face. She never laughed and never played with other children. . . . they did not like her, picked on her and called her 'crazy.' . . . The girl's school record supplies interesting objective evidence of a beginning mental disease—all A's in the 4th grade, A's and B's in 5-A, B's and C's in 5-B, and C's and D's in the 6th grade, pointing to the increasing severity of the process" (pp. 215–216).

Kasanin and Veo's Group V included those subjects who were "typical 'nobodies' in school, and no matter how many teachers were interviewed, they had the greatest difficulty in recalling them. These children were so seclusive, and made so very few friends, or no friends at all, that we could not find any chums of theirs, for the simple reason that they had no chums" (p. 221).

A19. "One half of the psychoses developed in children of Groups I and V; that is, as children they were either extremely odd or queer, or else usually shy, passive and withdrawn. These two groups ought to be of special significance to mental hygienists because they are comparatively easily recognized" (Kasanin & Veo, p. 226).

A20. R. Lay (1938): "Vogt wrote that mental illnesses can thus occur before puberty, which resemble dementia praecox so much in symptomatology, progress and general character, that they must be considered early forms of this disease; katatonic, hebephrenic and paranoid conditions may be distinguished; sometimes the disease is grafted upon feeblemindedness; in some cases peculiarities of behavior are to be seen before the onset, and occasionally improvement or remission takes place. His conclusions thus agree in general with the features of the disease in adults" (p. 107).

Lay also reviews the paper of Ssucharewa (1932) which claimed that "in 107 cases, aged 7 to 17, there were 25 under 13 years of age. Most of the latter were catatonic, although a few were hebephrenic in type. The type of illness occurring before puberty is usually chronic in its course, only 7 of the 25 have an acute onset. This material shows also that age plays some part in determining prognosis, post-pubertal schizophrenia usually have a better outcome" (p. 108).

Lay also quotes Corberi's (1930) analysis: "Dementia praecocissima is a prepubertal schizophrenia with an unfavorable prognosis, and consists of mixed functional and organic cerebral symptoms, with a catatonic and hebephrenic type of course. Speech degenerates to mannerisms and stereotypies; the dementia fluctuates and remissions occur. In dementia infantilis the speech upset is an organic aphasis, the dementia is lasting and final, the course rapidly progressive" (p. 129).

A21. J. L. Despert (1940): "The children's answers to questions regarding the reality of their phantasied situations fall into 3 categories: (1) denial of character of reality; (2) evasion; (3) reiteration with apparent belief. . . . The latter category, containing the smallest number of responses, included those responses in which a strong emotional component is evident, chiefly fears, but also wishes" (p. 211).

A22. "In our group of normal children it is not among the most imaginative children that pseudo-hallucinatory or pseudo-delusional experiences were most frequently encountered. Girl No. 11, with probably the richest phantasy life . . . never fails to assert her lack of belief in the "reality" of her phantasies. . . . On the other hand, Boy No. 27 . . . the only child among the thirty children . . . who could be described as showing borderline behavior—that is, poor social adaptation associated with preoccupation, anxiety in response to pseudo-hallucinations such as visualizing insects, destructiveness, mild touching compulsion—is amongst the least imaginative . . ." (Despert, 1940, p. 208).

A23. J. L. Despert (1947): "For instance, a normal child might, in fun, put a wastebasket on his head; but he, as well as the observer, is fully aware that this activity is carried out in fun; whereas the 9 year old schizophrenic boy, John N., doing the same thing, walks about solemnly, with no expressed or hidden intention of fun" (pp. 683-684).

A24. "For conformism is so characteristic of the young normal child . . . with all of the individuality of the young child's behavior, it is readily recognized that children in a group spontaneously conform to certain patterns of behavior which the schizophrenic child ignores" (Despert, 1947, p. 684).

A25. "The speech peculiarities as they involve voice, pitch, rhythm and modulation . . . are probably related to the inadequacy of the emotional tone of speech content" (Despert, 1947, p. 685).

A26. C. Bradley (1947): "In searching for important objective evidence of the presence of psychoses in children, the following three plans of study have been pursued: (1) behavior symptoms capable of description in children presumably psychotic at the time of observation have been investigated and evaluated; (2) past histories of children known to be psychotic have been searched for reports of their earliest maladjustment; and (3) a search has been made for reliable notes written on the spot in diaries or bably books describing step by step the growth and reactions of children who later became psychotic, so that the evolution of a psychosis, in terms used by parents to describe what they have seen, might become available" (p. 531).

A27. L. Kanner (1949): "Not one of the 55 patients studied has had in his infancy any disease or physical injury to which his behavior could be possibly ascribed by any stretch of the imagination. . . . On the whole, the children are well formed, well developed, rather slender, and attractive" (p. 420).

A28. "It has been customary to assign to Heller's disease a place among the forms of Childhood Schizophrenia. Corberi in Italy did a biopsy of cortical tissue in two cases and found wide areas of ganglion cell degeneration and shrinkage of the cell processes. This was fully verified in two cases of my own observation. It is therefore appropriate to separate Heller's disease from the schizophrenias and to align it with the organic degenerative disorders akin to the Tay-Sachs disease group."

"Early infantile autism bears no resemblance to Heller's disease or to any other organic condition. Heller's disease has a definite onset; the child impresses people as feeling and being sick. In fact, Zappert counted this initial malaise, or 'Krankheitsgefuhl,' among the essential features of Heller's disease. . . . Our autistic children did not go through such a prodromal stage. . . . Even those patients who have withdrawn to the point of functional idiocy or imbecility show, especially in their behavior with puzzles and form boards, residual oases of planned mental activity which should deter one from thinking in terms of a degenerative organic process" (Kanner, 1949, p. 417).

A29. "I have seen word-deaf children who were shy, apprehensive, lacking in spontaneity, pathetically bewildered, and insecure. But they all responded promptly to gestures, were keenly sensitive to physiognomies, and had a definite relation to their mothers, mostly one of clinging dependence. None showed the isolation, obsessiveness, and fragmentation of interests typical of early infantile autism. Certainly, there are enough autistic children who have amazingly large vocabularies. . . . Even some of the mute children have astounded their parents by uttering well-formed sentences in emergency situations. . . . Those who eventually begin to talk give evidence that during the silent period they have accumulated a considerable store of readily available linguistic material" (Kanner, 1949, pp. 417–418).

A30. In his 1949 paper, Kanner quotes from a thoughtful letter he received from Louise Despert: "If, leaving aside the nature of etiology, we agree on the descriptive definition of schizophrenia as a withdrawal of affect from reality, then where are we going to draw the line? At adolescence? During pre-adolescent years? During childhood? In early childhood years? Obviously the symptoms which are an expression of the withdrawal of affect must vary according to the developmental level and the structure of personality at various age levels. It cannot be accidentally that the symptoms described by you have an almost word-for-word similarity with the symptoms which I, for instance, have described regarding the language-sign and language function, the fear of noise, the compulsive acts, the need for things to be the same, etc." (Kanner, 1949, p. 419).

A31. "Some of these parents have been able to rear other children who did not withdraw. . . . furthermore, I have seen parent couples who answered the above characterization to the fullest extent, yet whose offspring, far from withdrawing autistically, responded with restless aggressiveness."

"Do not the personalities of the parents indicate that there are milder degrees of detachment and obsessiveness which enable a person to function and even gain a certain type of success in a nonpsychotic existence?" (Kanner, 1949, p. 426).

A32. B. W. Richards (1951): ". . . mental grade as being determined where possible, by the results of mental tests; where not, by ability to read and write and carry on a conversation."

"Dementia is considered to be absent if the patient conforms to basic social demands, such as clean toilet habits, washing, dressing and feeding, answering when spoken to and giving an account of himself in conversation. Its presence is recognized, apart from failure to adapt in above-mentioned respects, by irrelevant, incoherent or mumbling answers, with wandering of attention, when addressed. More severe dementia is shown by mutism, giggling, echolalia or moving away when approached, showing complete absence of any attempt to conform to the important social requirement of maintaining contact with fellow men. Incontinence and refusal to wash and dress are evidence of extreme dementia" (pp. 291–292).

A33. "That a patient may demonstrate schizoid traits so soon as infant behavior is sufficiently differentiated to reveal them is certain, and this presents no diagnostic problem if the tendency is not pronounced enough to hinder mental maturation in early life, but if it is so severe as to prevent the development of subject/object relations during the first year of life, it may be impossible to know if the schizophrenic process is acting alone or not" (Richards, 1951, p. 299).

A34. "Age does not seem to play an important part in determining the intensity of the disease process; that is to say, with onset at any given age, the disease may be mild or severe."

"Age acts as a limiting factor, for a psychosis which prevents mental progress entirely will result in a greater degree of defect the earlier the stage of mental development" (Richards, 1951, p. 305).

A35. "The degree of mental defect is, therefore, determined by intensity at least as much as by age of onset. The degree of dementia is also decided by intensity rather than by age, for there is no special tendency of schizophrenia of early onset to proceed to severe dementia, judging by our cases and by reports in the literature" (Richards, 1951, p. 305).

A36. "Body build may also be a prognostic aid. Three of our patients were markedly leptosomatic, with long slim hands and sharp, delicate features, small bones and slender build. All three showed hebephrenic features and were moderately demented" (Richards, 1951, p. 307).

REFERENCES

This list of references includes only papers and books that are referred to in this book and are, with two exceptions, available in the English language. The list in no way represents a comprehensive bibliography on the subject of childhood schizophrenia. For such a comprehensive review, the reader is referred to Goldfarb and Dorsen (1956) and Fish and Ritvo (1979).

Alexander, H. Insanity in children. *Journal of the American Medical Association 21*: 511–519, 1893.

American Psychiatric Association. *Diagnostic and statistical manual of mental disorders* (3rd ed.). American Psychiatric Association Press, Washington, DC, 1980.

American Psychiatric Association. *Diagnostic and statistical manual of mental disorders* (3rd ed., rev.). American Psychiatric Association Press, Washington, DC, 1987.

Angus, L. R. Schizophrenia and schizoid conditions in students in a special school. *American Journal of Mental Deficiency 53*: 227–238, 1948.

Anthony, E. J. An aetiological approach to the diagnosis of psychosis in childhood. *Acta Paedopsychiatrica 25*: 89–96, 1958.

Asarnow, J., & Goldstein, M. Schizophrenia during early adolescence and adulthood: A developmental perspective on risk research. *Clinical Psychology Review 6*: 211–235, 1986.

Bakwin, H. Emotional disturbances in children. *Yearbook of Pediatrics*: 422–424, 1950a.

Bakwin, H. Psychologic aspects of pediatrics: Childhood schizophrenia. *Journal of Pediatrics 37*: 416–426, 1950b.

Bakwin, H. Etiology of behavior disorders in children. *Postgraduate Medicine 9*: 260–265, 1951.

Bender, L. Childhood schizophrenia. *Nervous Child 1*: 138–140, 1941–1942.

Bender, L. Childhood schizophrenia: A clinical study of 100 schizophrenic children. *American Journal of Orthopsychiatry 17*: 40–56, 1947.

Bender, L. The life course of schizophrenic children. *Biological Psychiatry 2*: 165–172, 1970.

Bender, L., & Freedman, A. M. A study of the first three years in the maturation of schizophrenic children. *Quarterly Journal of Child Behavior 4*: 245–272, 1952.

Bender, L., Freedman, A. M., Grugett, A. E., Jr., & Helme, W. Schizophrenia in childhood, a confirmation of the diagnosis. *Transactions of the American Neurological Association 77*: 67–73, 1952.

Bennett, S., & Klein, H. R. Childhood schizophrenia: 30 years later. *American Journal of Psychiatry 122*: 1121–1124, 1966.

Bergman, M., Waller, H., & Marchand, J. Schizophrenic reactions during childhood in mental defectives. *Psychiatric Quarterly 25*: 294–333, 1951.

Bleuler, E. *Dementia praecox or the group of schizophrenias* (J. Zinkin, Trans.). International Universities Press, New York, 1950. (Original work published in German in 1911)

Bowman, K. M., & Kasanin, J. Constitutional schizophrenia. *American Journal of Psychiatry 13*: 645–658, 1933.

Bradley, C. *Schizophrenia in childhood*. Macmillan, New York, 1941.

Bradley, C. Early evidence of psychoses in children, with special reference to schizophrenia. *Journal of Pediatrics 30*: 529–540, 1947.

Brierre de Boismont, M. On the insanity of early life. *Journal of Psychological Medicine and Mental Pathology 10*: 622–638, 1857.

Browne, J. C. Psychical diseases of early life. *Journal of Mental Science 6*: 284–320, 1859–1860.

Bruininks, R. H. *Bruininks–Oseretsky Test of Motor Proficiency: Examiner's manual*. American Guidance Service, Circle Pines, MN, 1978.

Burr, C. W. Insanity at puberty. *Journal of the American Medical Association 45*: 36–39, 1905.

Burr, C. W. The mental disorders of childhood. *American Journal of Psychiatry 5*: 145–161, 1925.

Cameron, N. Reasoning, regression, and communication in schizophrenics. *Psychological Monographs 50*(1, Whole No. 221), 1938.

Canavan, M. M., & Clark, R. The mental health of 463 children from dementia-praecox stock. *Mental Hygiene 7*: 137–148, 1923a.

Canavan, M. M., & Clark, R. The mental health of 581 offspring of non-psychotic parents. *Mental Hygiene 7*: 770–778, 1923b.

Cantor, S. Resolved: There exists an atropinic agent in vivo. *Medical Hypotheses 6*: 801–805, 1980.

Cantor, S. *The schizophrenic child*. Eden Press, Montreal, Quebec, 1982.

Cantor, S., Evans, J., Pearce, J., & Pezzot-Pearce, T. Childhood schizophrenia: Present but not accounted for. *American Journal of Psychiatry 139*(6): 758–762, 1982.

Cantor, S., & Kestenbaum, C. Psychotherapy with schizophrenic children. *Journal of the American Academy of Child Psychiatry 25*(5): 623–630, 1986.

Cantor, S., Pearce, J., Pezzot-Pearce, T., & Evans, J. The group of hypotonic schizophrenics. *Schizophrenia Bulletin 7*: 1–11, 1981.

Cantor, S., Trevenen, C., Postuma, R., Dueck, R., & Fjeldsted, B. Is childhood schizophrenia a cholinergic disease? *Archives of General Psychiatry 37*: 658–667, 1980.

Childers, A. T. A study of some schizoid children. *Mental Hygiene 15*: 106–134, 1931.

Clouston, T. S. *Clinical lectures on mental disease.* Henry C. Lea's Son, Philadelphia, 1884.

Conolly, J. Juvenile insanity. *American Journal of Insanity 18:* 395–403, 1861–1862.

Corberi, G. *Infanzia Anormale 3:* 201–211, 1930.

Courtney, J. W. The youthful psychopath. *Boston Medical and Surgical Journal 164:* 219–222, 1911.

Creak, M. Schizophrenia syndrome in childhood: Further progress report of a working party. *Developmental Medicine and Child Neurology 6:* 530–535, 1964.

Darr, G. C., & Worden, F. G. Case report twenty-eight years after an infantile autistic disorder. *American Journal of Orthopsychiatry 21:* 559–570, 1951.

De Sanctis, S. Sopra alcuna varieta della demenza precoce. *Rivista Sperimentale di Freniatria e Medicina Legale delle Alienazioni Mentale:* 141–165, 1906.

Despert, J. L. Schizophrenia in children. *Psychiatric Quarterly 12:* 366–371, 1938.

Despert, J. L. A comparative study of thinking in schizophrenic children and in children of preschool age. *American Journal of Psychiatry 97:* 189–213, 1940.

Despert, J. L. The early recognition of childhood schizophrenia. *Medical Clinics of North America, Pediatrics 31*(3): 680–687, 1947.

Dillion, W. R., & Goldstein, M. *Multivariate analysis—methods and applications.* Wiley, New York, 1984.

Farnell, F. J. The psychopathic child. *Archives of Pediatrics 31:* 684–690, 1914.

Feingold, M., & Bossert, W. Normal values for selected physical parameters: An aid to syndrome delineation. In *Birth defects: Original articles series,* ed. by D. Bergsma (Vol. 10, p. 13). National Foundation–March of Dimes, White Plains, NY, 1974.

Fish, B. Neurobiologic antecedents of schizophrenia in children. *Archives of General Psychiatry 34:* 1297–1313, 1977.

Fish, B. Antecedents of an "Acute" Schizophrenic Break. *Journal of the American Academy of Child Psychiatry 25*(5): 595–600, 1986.

Fish, B., & Ritvo, E. Psychoses of childhood. In *Basic handbook of child psychiatry,* ed. by J. Noshpitz (Vol. 2, pp. 249–304). Basic Books, New York, 1979.

Fish, B., Shapiro, T., Campbell, M., & Wile, R. A classification of schizophrenic children under five years. *American Journal of Psychiatry 124:* 1415–1423, 1968.

Freeman, T., Cameron, J. L., & McGhie, A. *Chronic schizophrenia.* International Universities Press, New York, 1973.

Freud, A. *The writing of Anna Freud,* Vol. 2: *The ego and the mechanisms of defense.* International Universities Press, New York, 1965a.

Freud, A. *The writing of Anna Freud,* Vol. 6: *Normality and pathology in childhood: Assessments of development.* International Universities Press, New York, 1965b.

Goddard, H. H. The problem of the psychopathic child. *American Journal of Insanity 77*: 511–516, 1920.

Goldfarb, W. *Childhood schizophrenia*. Harvard University Press, Cambridge, MA, 1961.

Goldfarb, W. Factors in the development of schizophrenic children: An approach to subclassification. In *The origins of schizophrenia*, ed. by J. Romano. Excerpta Medica Foundation, New York, 1967.

Goldfarb, W., & Dorsen, M. M. *Annotated bibliography of childhood schizophrenia*. Basic Books, New York, 1956.

Goodhart, S. P. Atypical children: The etiological factors in their production. *New York Medical Journal 97*: 750–755, 1913.

Harms, E. Two case histories; Reports from two mothers. *Nervous Child 10*: 19–35, 1952.

Hollingshead, A. B., & Redlich, F. C. Social stratification and psychiatric disorders. *American Sociological Review 18*: 163–169, 1953.

Holmes, C. Insanity in children. *New York Medical Journal 95*: 283–284, 1912.

Hulse, W. Dementia infantalis. *Journal of Nervous and Mental Disease 119*: 471–477, 1954. (Translation of Heller's 1930 paper)

Hyde, G. E. Recognition of prepsychotic children by group mental tests. *American Journal of Psychiatry 2*: 43–48, 1922–1923.

Kanner, L. *Child psychiatry* (1st ed.). C. C. Thomas, Springfield, IL, 1935.

Kanner, L. Autistic disturbances of affective contact. *Nervous Child 2*: 217–250, 1942–1943.

Kanner, L. *Child psychiatry* (2nd ed.). C. C. Thomas, Springfield, IL, 1948.

Kanner, L. Problems of nosology and psychodynamics of early infantile autism. *American Journal of Orthopsychiatry 19*: 416–426, 1949.

Kasanin, J., & Kaufman, M. R. A study of the functional psychoses in childhood. *American Journal of Psychiatry 9*: 307–384, 1929.

Kasanin, J., & Veo, L. A study of the school adjustments of children who later in life become psychotic. *American Journal of Orthopsychiatry 2*: 212–230, 1932.

Kernberg, O. *Borderline conditions and pathological narcissism*. Aronson, New York, 1975.

Kraepelin, E. *Dementia praecox and paraphrenia* (R. M. Barclay, Trans.; G. M. Robertson, Ed.). Robert E. Krieger, Huntington, NY, 1971.

Lampron, E. M. Children of schizophrenic parents. *Mental Hygiene 17*: 82–91, 1933.

Langer, E. A case of suspected schizophrenia in a three year old. *Nervous Child 10*: 94–111, 1952.

Lay, R. A. Schizophrenia-like psychoses in young children. *Journal of Mental Science 84*: 105–133, 1938.

Lewis, D. D., Moy, E., Jackson, L. D., Aaronson, B. A., Restifo, N., Serra, S., & Simos, A. Biopsychosocial characteristics of children who later murder: A prospective study. *American Journal of Psychiatry 142*(10): 1161–1167, 1985.

Lourie, R. S., Pacella, B. L., & Piotrowski, Z. A. Studies on the prognosis in schizophrenic-like psychoses in children. *American Journal of Psychiatry* 99: 542–552, 1943.

Lurie, L. A., Tietz, E. B., & Hertzman, J. Functional psychoses in children. *American Journal of Psychiatry* 92: 1169–1184, 1936.

Marcus, J., Auerbach, J., Wilkonson, L., & Burack, C. M. Infants at risk for schizophrenia. *Archives of General Psychiatry* 38: 703–713, 1981.

Marcus, J., Hans, S. L., Mednick, S. A., Schulsinger, F., & Michelson, N. Neurological dysfunction in offspring of schizophrenics in Israel and Denmark. *Archives of General Psychiatry* 42: 753–761, 1985.

Maudsley, H. *The pathology of the mind.* Appleton, New York, 1880.

Mehr, H. M. The application of psychological tests and methods to schizophrenia in children. *Nervous Child* 10: 63–93, 1952.

Meyer, A. What do histories of insanity teach us concerning preventive mental hygiene during the years of school life? *Psychological Clinic* 2(4): 89–101, 1908.

Norman, E. Reality relationships of schizophrenic children. *British Journal of Medical Psychology* 27: 126–141, 1954.

Offord, D. R., & Cross, L. A. Behavioral antecedents of adult schizophrenia. *Archives of General Psychiatry* 21: 267–283, 1969.

O'Gorman, G. Psychosis as a cause of mental defect. *Journal of Mental Science* 100: 934–943, 1954.

Potter, H. W. Schizophrenia in children. *American Journal of Psychiatry* 12: 1253–1270, 1933.

Richards, B. W. Childhood schizophrenia and mental deficiency. *Journal of Mental Science* 97: 290–312, 1951.

Rosenthal, D., Wender, P. H., Kety, S. S., *et al.* Schizophrenics' offspring reared in adoptive homes. In *The transmission of schizophrenia,* ed. by D. Rosenthal & S. S. Kety. Pergamon Press, London, 1968.

Rutter, M. Childhood schizophrenia reconsidered. *Journal of Autism and Childhood Schizophrenia* 2: 315–337, 1972.

Schreiber, F. R. *The shoemaker.* Simon and Schuster, New York, 1983.

Smith, J. A pediatrician views the trends in child psychiatry. *Archives of Pediatrics* 68: 477–487, 1951.

Spungen, D. *And I don't want to live this life.* Random House, New York, 1983.

Strecker, E. A. Psychoses and potential psychoses of childhood. *New York Medical Journal* 114: 209–211, 1921.

Tramer, M. Diary of a psychotic child (H. Bruch & F. Cottington, Trans.). *Nervous Child* 1: 232–249, 1941–1942.

Walker, S. H., & Duncan, D. B. Estimation of the probability of an event as a function of several independent variables. *Biometrica* 54: 169–179, 1967.

Wechsler, D. *Wechsler Adult Intelligent Scale.* The Psychological Corporation, New York, 1955.

Wechsler, D. *Wechsler Intelligence Scale for Children—Revised.* The Psychological Corporation, San Antonio, TX, 1974.

Wechsler, D., & Jaros, E. Schizophrenic patterns of WISC. *Journal of Clinical Psychology* 3: 288–291, 1965.

Wilson, L. *This stranger my son*. Longmans Canada Ltd., Toronto, Ontario, 1968.

Wing, L. *Autistic children*. Brunner/Mazel, New York, 1985.

Witmer, L. Orthogenic cases. 14. Don: A curable case of arrested development due to a fear psychosis the result of shock in a three-year-old infant. *The Psychological Clinic 13*: 97–111, 1920.

INDEX